Patient
Positioning

Patient Positioning

MARK J. SCHUBERT, R.T.(R)

Adjunct Faculty for The School of Radiologic Technology
at Tidewater Community College,
Virginia Beach, Virginia

SERIES EDITOR

STEWART C. BUSHONG, Sc.D., F.A.C.R., F.A.C.M.P.

Professor of Radiologic Science, Department of Radiology, Baylor College of Medicine, Houston, Texas

Illustrations by Holly R. Fischer, MFA
Ann Arbor, Michigan

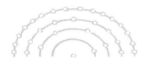

ESSENTIALS OF MEDICAL IMAGING SERIES

McGraw-Hill

Health Professions Division

New York St. Louis San Francisco Auckland Bogotá Caracas Lisbon London Madrid
Mexico City Milan Montreal New Delhi San Juan
Singapore Sydney Tokyo Toronto

McGraw-Hill
A Division of The McGraw·Hill Companies

Patient Positioning
Essentials of Medical Imaging Series
Copyright © 1999 by The McGraw-Hill Companies, Inc. All rights reserved.
Printed in the United States of America. Except as permitted under the
United States Copyright Act of 1976, no part of this publication may be
reproduced or distributed in any form or by any means, or stored in a data
base or retrieval system without the prior written permission of the publisher.

1 2 3 4 5 6 7 8 9 0   MALMAL   9 9 8

ISBN 0-07-058067-7

This book was set in Berkeley by V&M Graphics.
The editors were John J. Dolan and Peter McCurdy.
The production supervisor was Heather A. Barry.
The text designer was José R. Fonfrias.
The cover designer was Robert Freese.
Malloy Lithographing, Inc. was printer and binder.

This book is printed on acid-free paper.

Visit The McGraw-Hill Health Professions Website at http://www.mghmedical.com

Cataloging-in-Publication data is on file for this title at the Library of Congress.

Contents

CHAPTER 8

GASTROINTESTINAL TRACT   69

CHAPTER 9

URINARY SYSTEM   77

CHAPTER 10

SPECIAL EXAMINATIONS   81

APPENDIX A

GLOSSARY   89

APPENDIX B

BIBLIOGRAPHY   93

APPENDIX C

ANSWERS TO PRACTICE QUESTIONS   95

Preface

This book is intended to be used as a positioning study guide in preparation for the National Registry Examination for Radiologic Technologists (aka the ARRT examination). It is also written in a way to help refresh positioning skills and challenge the mind of a seasoned radiologic technologist.

The chapters in this book are concise, loaded with useful information, and followed by registry-style review questions. The glossary will provide a quick reference for any unfamiliar terms used throughout the text.

It is my hope that this book will provide a helping hand for what is otherwise a stressful examination preparation process.

Acknowledgments

This book is in part dedicated to my loving and ever supportive wife, Sheila. She is my best friend and partner in life. Without Sheila's valuable guidance, understanding, and tolerance (especially following a "burning the midnight oil session"), this book would not be a reality. Thanks! Sheila.

There have been many people during my x-ray career who have helped develop my skills and inspired me to reach for the stars in career potential. I am forever grateful to these individuals and would like to take this opportunity to acknowledge their influence.

First and foremost, I would like to thank the educators and staff at Peninsula Hospital for introducing me to the exciting world of x-ray science. Special thanks to Betsy, Carole, "Reg", Donna, Andy, and Cheryl.

I would also like to thank my mentors Kim Burford-Utley and Judith Cook for the encouragement and opportunities provided to me while "under their wings." I am a better person, technologist and educator because of you two wonderful ladies. Special Thanks! Judy and Kim.

I would like to thank my first English Professor for unveiling my creativity and writing talent. Without his helping hand (red pencil) and words of praise I would not have been bold enough to publish. Thank You, Thank You, Thank You!

I would lastly like to thank all the folks at McGraw-Hill and my friend Stewart Bushong for making this an enjoyable and comfortable venture. Thanks everyone!

Patient Positioning

Introduction and Terminology

GENERAL

- A **radiograph** is an x-ray film with a manifest anatomical image.

- **Radiography** is the art of producing radiographs.

- The **radiographic procedure** includes a variety of functions leading to a diagnostic image product.

- Radiographs are typically displayed as if the patient were standing before the viewer in the anatomical position.

- The **anatomical position** refers to an erect body, with feet together, arms at the sides, and palms facing forward.

- The form of the body determines the general size, shape, and position of the internal organs. The term **body habitus** is used to describe different body forms. The **hypersthenic** body type is of massive build, with organs having a high, transverse placement and usually a short, broad shape. The **sthenic** habitus is the average body shape. **Hyposthenic** and **asthenic** are smaller, thinner body types typically having long, narrow organs with low placement.

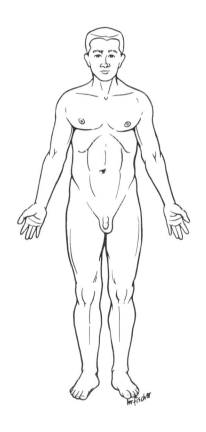

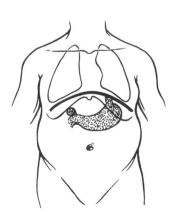

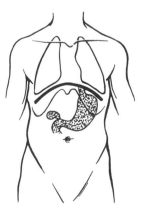

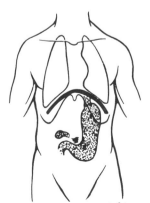

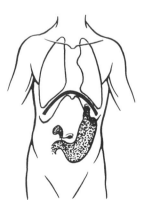

Hypersthenic habitus   Sthenic habitus   Hyposthenic habitus   Asthenic habitus

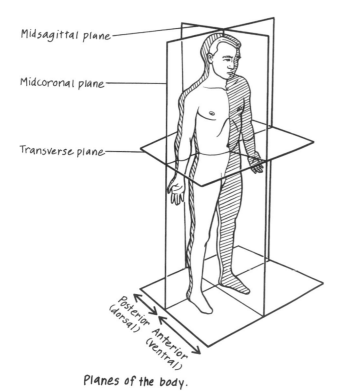

Planes of the body.

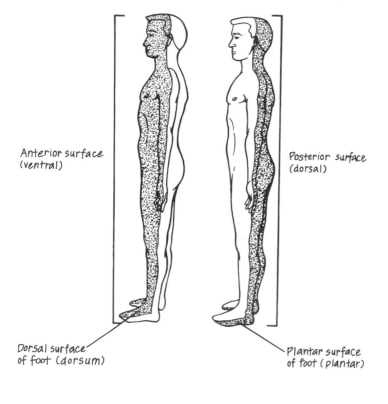

BODY PLANES

- There are three fundamental planes by which the body can be divided.

- The **sagittal plane** divides the body vertically into right and left portions. In addition, the **midsagittal plane (MSP)** is a midline plane dividing the body into *equal* right and left halves.

- The **coronal** or **frontal plane** is a vertical plane dividing the body into front (anterior) and back (posterior) portions. In addition, the **midcoronal** or **midfrontal plane** provides *equal* division of front and back portions.

- The **transverse** or **axial plane** is a horizontal plane dividing the body into superior and inferior portions.

BODY SURFACES AND LANDMARKS

- **Anterior** or **ventral** refers to the front or forward part of the body.

- The back of the body or of a body part is commonly called **posterior** or **dorsal**.

- The palm of the hand is known as the **palmar** surface.

- The sole (bottom) of the foot is called the **plantar** surface, and the top of the foot is termed the **dorsum**.

- The **mastoid tip** is found at about the level of C1.

- The **thyroid cartilage** is located at approximately C5.

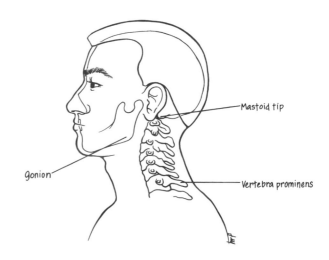

- The seventh cervical vertebra can be located by palpating the long spinous process known as the **vertebra prominens**.

- The **sternal (manubrial) notch** indicates the level of T2 and T3.

- The radiographer can use the **inferior angle** of the **scapula** to locate the level of T7.

- The **xiphoid tip** marks the location (level) of T10.

- The level of the **umbilicus** indicates where L4 and the most superior aspect of the iliac crest (IC) are located.

- The level of sacral segment 1 can be found by palpating for the **anterior superior iliac spine** (ASIS).

- The coccyx is located at the same level as the **pubic symphysis** and the **greater trochanters**.

BODY POSITIONS AND PROJECTIONS

- **Position** refers to the manner in which the patient is placed in relation to the film or surrounding space.

- The direction or path of the x-ray beam as it passes through the patient is commonly known as the **projection**.

- The general body position in which the patient is lying on his or her back is the **supine position**.

- The opposite of the supine position, where the patient lies facing downward, is the **prone position**.

- The **erect position** is the upright (seated or standing) position.

- The term **recumbent** means that the patient is lying down in any position.

- When the patient is recumbent with the head lower than the feet, he or she is said to be in the **Trendelenburg position**.

- In a **Fowler's position**, the patient's head is higher than the feet.

- The **lithotomy position** places the patient supine, with knees and hip flexed, thighs abducted, and legs placed on supports.

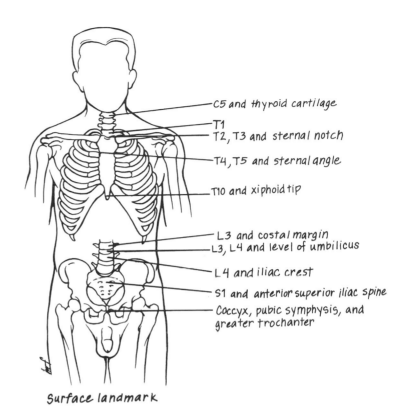

C5 and thyroid cartilage
T1
T2, T3 and sternal notch
T4, T5 and sternal angle
T10 and xiphoid tip
L3 and costal margin
L3, L4 and level of umbilicus
L4 and iliac crest
S1 and anterior superior iliac spine
Coccyx, pubic symphysis, and greater trochanter

Surface landmark

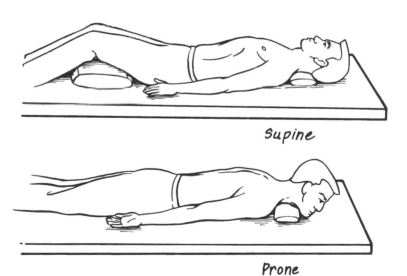

Supine

Prone

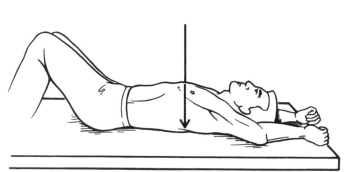

AP (anteroposterior) projection

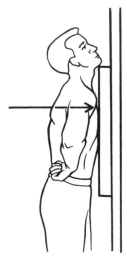 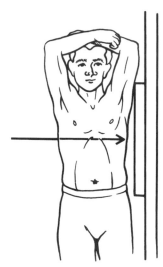

PA (posteranterior
projection

Left lateral
position

- **Frontal projections** describe the manner in which the x-ray beam enters and exits the body. Examples include
    1. Anteroposterior (AP) projection: the x-ray beam enters the front surface and exits the back surface.
    2. Posteroanterior (PA) projection: the x-ray beam enters the back surface and exits the front surface.

- The **lateral position** provides a side view of a body part and is specifically named by the side closest to the film.

- The **oblique position** involves rotation of a body part so that neither a frontal nor a lateral image is produced.

- Some examples of oblique positions include
    1. Left posterior oblique (LPO): the left posterior part of the body is closest to the film.
    2. Right posterior oblique (RPO): the right posterior part of the body is closest to the film.
    3. Left anterior oblique (LAO): the left anterior part of the body is closest to the film.
    4. Right anterior oblique (RAO): the right anterior part of the body is closest to the film.

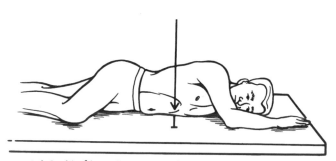

LAO (left anterior oblique) position

- A position in which the patient is lying down (recumbent) and the central ray is parallel to the horizon is known as the **decubitus position**. There are lateral, ventral (prone), and dorsal (supine) decubitus positions.

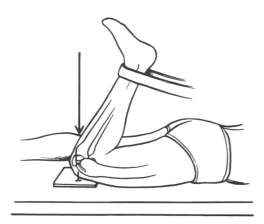

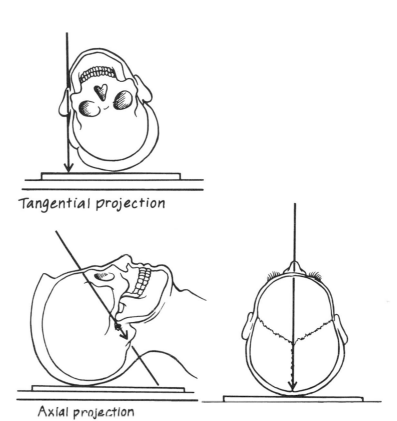

Tangential projection

Axial projection

- In a **tangential projection** the central ray skims the body part to project that part free of super-imposition.

- When the central ray is angled along the long axis of a body part, it is said to have an **axial** projection.

- Certain radiologic procedures are named after individuals. These individuals have developed **methods** that can be used to demonstrate a specific anatomical part (e.g., the Waters, Law, and Caldwell methods).

MOVEMENT TERMS

- To **flex** a joint is to bend it, and to extend a joint is to straighten it out.

- **Dorsiflexion** means flexing the top of the foot upward, and **plantar flexion** refers to extending the foot downward.

- **Eversion** describes outward movement (stress), and **inversion** describes inward movement (stress).

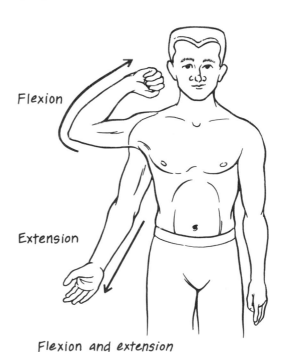

Flexion

Extension

Flexion and extension

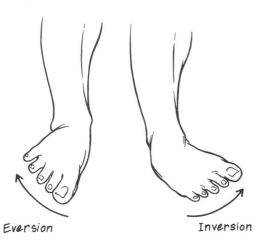

Eversion   Inversion

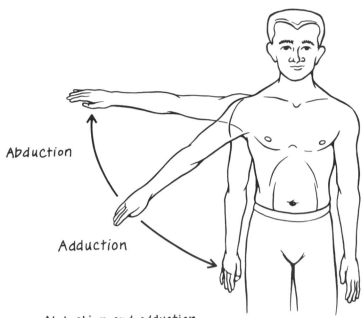

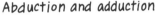

Abduction and adduction

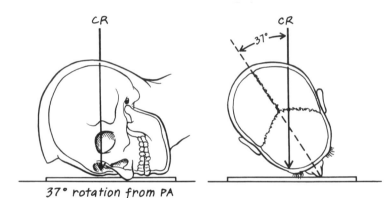

37° rotation from PA

- **Medial rotation** is movement of a body part inward (medially), and **lateral rotation** is movement of a body part outward (laterally).

- To **abduct** a body part is to draw it away from the body's midline, and to **adduct** a body part is to draw it closer to the body's midline.

- **Supination** places the hand supine or palm up, and **pronation** places the hand with the palm down (prone).

- When a body part is *not* in alignment with the long axis of the body, it is said to be **tilted**.

- **Rotation** is the turning of a body part from the frontal position while maintaining alignment with the body's long axis.

- The term **caudad (caudal)** refers to a location away from the head of the patient. Caudad can be a direction in which the central ray is pointed away from the patient's head.

- **Cephalad (cephalic)** refers to body parts toward the head or to a central ray direction pointed toward the head.

Chapter 1 Practice Questions

1. Turning a body part inward is termed
   a. extension.
   b. flexion.
   c. inversion.
   d. eversion.

2. A vertical plane that divides the body into anterior and posterior portions is called a
   a. sagittal plane.
   b. transverse plane.
   c. squamosal plane.
   d. coronal plane.

3. The type of body form is called the

   a. Townes type.
   b. body habitus.
   c. anatomical form.
   d. simple form.

4. When the head is in the PA position, it is

   a. extended.
   b. supinated.
   c. abducted.
   d. pronated.

5. The dorsum of the foot is the

   a. lateral side.
   b. superior aspect.
   c. medial side.
   d. inferior aspect.

6. The term *position* describes

   a. a radiation path.
   b. patient placement.
   c. a body plane.
   d. body size.

7. Terms referring to the front body surface include

   1. anterior   a. only 1.
   2. posterior.   b. only 2
   3. ventral.   c. 2 and 3
                        d. 1 and 3

8. The body plane dividing the body into right and left equal portions is the

   a. midsagittal.
   b. midcoronal.
   c. midaxillary.
   d. midtransverse.

9. Which body position refers to standing erect with the palms forward?

   a. anatomical
   b. prone
   c. supine
   d. lateral

10. The ASIS is at the level of

    a. L3.
    b. L4.
    c. S2.
    d. S1.

11. The ventral decubitus position is similar to the

    a. supine position.
    b. prone position.
    c. lateral position.
    d. erect position.

12. A rotated body position that is not frontal or lateral is termed
    a. axial.
    b. tangential.
    c. oblique.
    d. decubitus.

13. A PA oblique position can correspond to

    | 1. RAO. | a. 1 and 2 |
    | 2. RPO. | b. 2 and 3 |
    | 3. LPO. | c. 1 and 4 |
    | 4. LAO. | d. 3 and 4 |

14. Turning the foot outward is an example of
    a. inversion.
    b. flexion.
    c. pronation.
    d. eversion.

15. A large person with high, transverse organs is classified as
    a. sthenic.
    b. hyposthenic.
    c. hypersthenic.
    d. asthenic.

16. The L4 vertebral body corresponds to the level of the
    a. gonion.
    b. IC.
    c. sacrum.
    d. mentum.

17. The lateral decubitus position is an example of
    a. a lateral projection.
    b. a frontal projection.
    c. an oblique projection.
    d. a tangential projection.

18. The movement of a body part toward the body's midline is called
    a. prone.
    b. abduction.
    c. adduction.
    d. caudal.

19. The term *projection* describes
    a. a radiation path.
    b. patient placement.
    c. body size.
    d. a body plane.

20. Joint movement that increases the angle between the articulating bones is called
    a. eversion.
    b. extension.
    c. inversion.
    d. flexion.

21. A plane separating the body into upper and lower portions is a
    a. coronal plane.
    b. transverse plane.
    c. sagittal plane.
    d. frontal plane.

22. A term describing the front of the body is
    1. plantar.   a. 1 and 2
    2. ventral.   b. 3 and 4
    3. dorsal.   c. 1 and 4
    4. anterior.   d. 2 and 4

23. The thyroid cartilage is located at the level of
    a. C1.
    b. C7.
    c. C5.
    d. T1.

24. A patient positioned with the head higher than the feet is in which position?
    a. recumbent
    b. Fowler's
    c. lithotomy
    d. Trendelenburg

25. The dorsal decubitus position is most similar to the _____ position.
    a. prone
    b. supine
    c. lateral
    d. axial

26. When the central ray is directed toward the head, it is said to have a
    a. caudad angle.
    b. axial angle.
    c. rotation angle.
    d. cephalad angle.

27. Supinating the hand places the palm
    a. down.
    b. up.
    c. lateral.
    d. tilted.

28. An AP projection with the left side rotated closest to the film is called

    a. RAO.
    b. LAO.
    c. RPO.
    d. LPO.

29. The central ray projection that describes skimming a body part is called

    a. tangential.
    b. axial.
    c. decubitus.
    d. lateral.

30. This term describes a patient lying down in any position.

    a. PA
    b. recumbent
    c. lateral
    d. AP

Upper Extremity

FINGERS

- The correct central ray location in imaging digits 2 through 5 is at the proximal interphalangeal (PIP) joint.

- Fingers should be separated from each other so as to avoid the overlapping of soft tissue.

- The proper amount of obliquity used in the examination of a finger is 45°. The finger should remain parallel to the film when it is being placed in a 45° semiprone (PA) oblique position.

- The lateral finger (digit) position varies depending on the digit of interest. Digits 2 and 3 are positioned thumb side (lateral aspect) down, and digits 4 and 5 are positioned thumb side up.

- An AP projection of the first digit (thumb) is preferred because it reduces the object-image distance (OID).

- The central ray location for any position or projection of the thumb is at the first metacarpophalangeal (MP) joint.

- An oblique position of the thumb is achieved when the hand is placed palm down on the cassette as in a PA hand position.

- The entire first metacarpal is seen when the thumb is imaged.

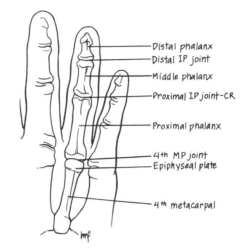

Distal phalanx
Distal IP joint
Middle phalanx
Proximal IP joint-CR
Proximal phalanx
4th MP joint
Epiphyseal plate
4th metacarpal

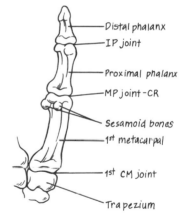

Distal phalanx
IP joint
Proximal phalanx
MP joint-CR
Sesamoid bones
1st metacarpal
1st CM joint
Trapezium

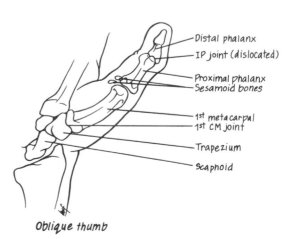

Distal phalanx
IP joint (dislocated)
Proximal phalanx
Sesamoid bones
1st metacarpal
1st CM joint
Trapezium
Scaphoid

Oblique thumb

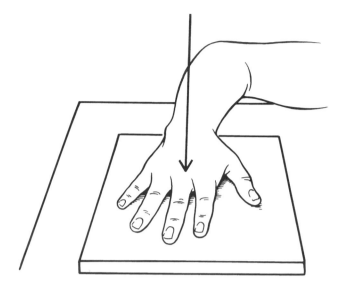

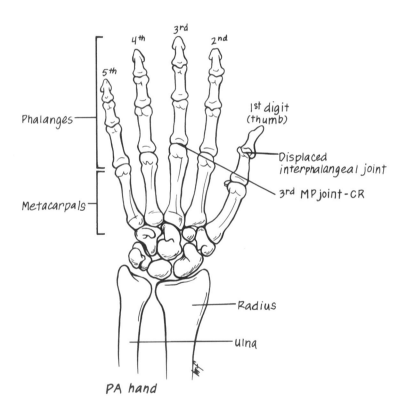

PA hand

HAND

- The average-size hand fits on an 8×10 film lengthwise or 10×12 crosswise divided in half.

- In a PA hand position the hand is pronated so that the palmar surface rests on the cassette.

- The central ray is directed toward the third MP joint when the PA, AP, or oblique hand is being imaged.

- A PA projection of the hand demonstrates an oblique image of the first digit (thumb).

- The hand is rotated semiprone 45° with the ulnar side down for a proper oblique position.

- When imaging the hand laterally, place the central ray perpendicular to the second through fifth MP joints.

- A hand is most commonly positioned laterally with the ulnar aspect down (against the film).

- The lateral hand can be optionally placed in a **fan lateral position**, which demonstrates the phalanges nearly free of superimposition, or in a **lateral in extension**, which demonstrates localization of foreign bodies and/or metacarpal fracture displacement.

- A bilateral AP 45° oblique position of the hands provides a helpful image for the diagnosis of rheumatoid arthritis. This imaging method is sometimes referred to as the **ball-catcher position**.

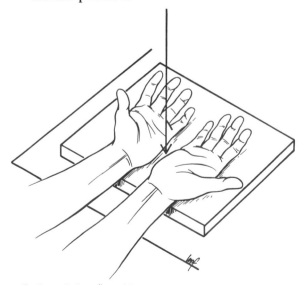

"Ball-catcher" position

WRIST

- When positioning the wrist for a PA projection instruct the patient to slightly flex the fingers in order to reduce the OID.

- The central ray location for a PA or AP wrist projection is at the midcarpal area.

- An AP projection of the wrist is superior to a PA projection for demonstrating carpal interspaces.

- The semiprone (45°) PA oblique wrist position (ulnar surface resting on the cassette) best demonstrates the carpals on the lateral side of the wrist, especially the navicular (scaphoid).

- The semisupine (45°) AP oblique wrist position (ulnar surface resting on the cassette) best demonstrates the carpals on the medial side of the wrist, especially the pisiform.

- An accurate true lateral position of the wrist is with the elbow flexed at 90° and the ulnar surface resting against the film.

- The carpal navicular (scaphoid) can be demonstrated without distortion (foreshortening) when imaged in a PA position with extreme ulnar flexion.

- The interspaces of the medial carpal bones are best demonstrated with the wrist in a PA position with extreme radial flexion.

- The **Stecher method** is an alternative position used to demonstrate the carpal navicular (scaphoid). This method requires either a 20° body part angulation or a 20° central ray angulation toward the elbow.

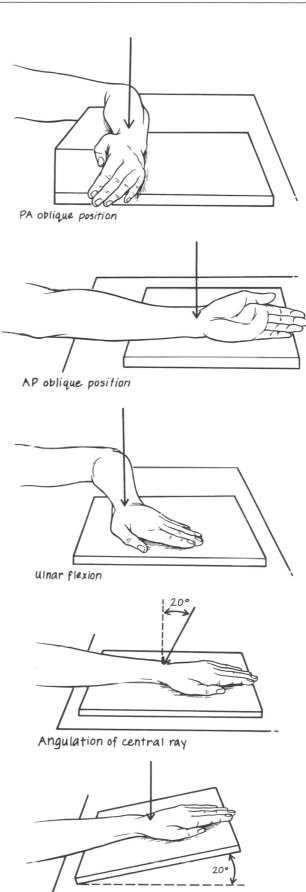

PA oblique position

AP oblique position

Ulnar flexion

Angulation of central ray

Angulation of part

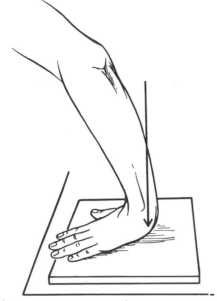

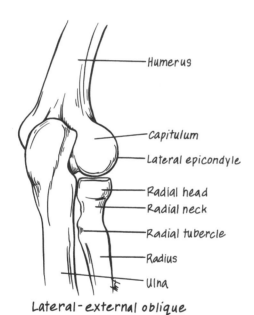

Superoinferior position

Humerus

Capitulum

Lateral epicondyle

Radial head

Radial neck

Radial tubercle

Radius

Ulna

Lateral-external oblique

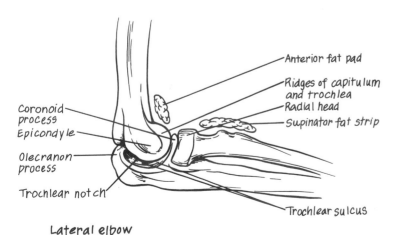

Coronoid process

Epicondyle

Olecranon process

Trochlear notch

Anterior fat pad

Ridges of capitulum and trochlea

Radial head

Supinator fat strip

Trochlear sulcus

Lateral elbow

- For the evaluation of **carpal tunnel syndrome**, a tangential position known as the **carpal canal (tunnel) position** is used. This position requires the wrist to be hyperextended (dorsiflexed) as far as possible with a central ray angle of 25 to 30° directed at 1 in. distal to the base of the third metacarpal.

- The dorsal aspect of the carpal bones can be imaged with the wrist in extreme palmar flexion, as in the **carpal bridge position**. This position requires a 45° central ray angle directed tangentially at the wrist joint.

FOREARM

- For an AP projection the forearm is positioned correctly when the humeral epicondyles are parallel to the film and the hand is supinated.

- A correct lateral forearm position is obtained with the elbow flexed 90°, humeral epicondyles perpendicular to the film, and the hand in a true lateral position with the thumb side up.

- The central ray is directed perpendicular to the midforearm for both AP and lateral images.

ELBOW

- An AP elbow projection is obtained with the arm fully extended and the hand supinated. The central ray should be directed toward the elbow joint.

- The AP 45° external (lateral) oblique position best demonstrates the radial head, neck, and tuberosity free of superimposition.

- To demonstrate the coronoid process in profile the patient is positioned in the AP 45° internal (medial) oblique position.

- The lateral elbow position requires the lower arm to be flexed 90° in order to properly demonstrate the olecranon process in profile.

- The humeral epicondyles must be perpendicular to the plane of the film and the hand placed in a true lateral position to obtain an accurate lateral elbow position.

- When the patient is unable to fully extend the elbow because of trauma, use the axiolateral projection (**Coyle method**) to demonstrate the radial head and/or the coronoid process.

- Varying the hand position while maintaining a true lateral elbow position effectively demonstrates the entire circumference of the radial head free of superimposition.

HUMERUS

- Include both the elbow and shoulder joints when the humerus is being imaged.

- Supinate the hand and adjust the humeral epicondyles to form a parallel relationship with the cassette for the AP humerus projection.

- An AP projection demonstrates the humeral head and greater tubercle in profile.

- The lateral humerus position requires medial rotation of the hand and arm to place the humeral epicondyles perpendicular to the cassette. This position demonstrates the lesser tubercle in profile.

- The proximal humerus can be imaged laterally by using the transthoracic position (**Lawrence method**). The epicondyles of the affected humerus are placed perpendicular to the film, and the unaffected arm is raised.

SHOULDER

- An AP external rotation shoulder position demonstrates the greater tubercle in profile laterally.

- The AP internal rotation shoulder position, with the humeral epicondyles perpendicular to the film, demonstrates the lesser tubercle in profile medially.

- For demonstration of the glenohumeral joint an inferosuperior axial position (Lawrence method) can be used. The patient is positioned supine, with the affected arm abducted 90° and a horizontal central ray directed through the axilla.

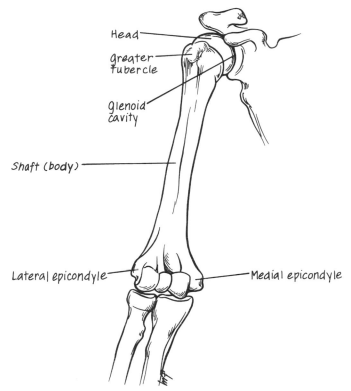

AP humerus

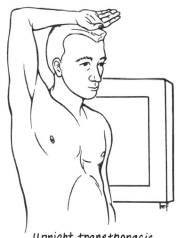

Upright transthoracic lateral position

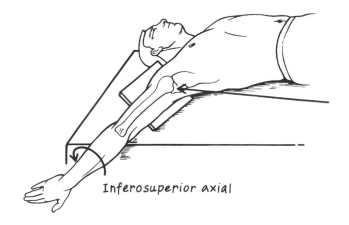

Inferosuperior axial

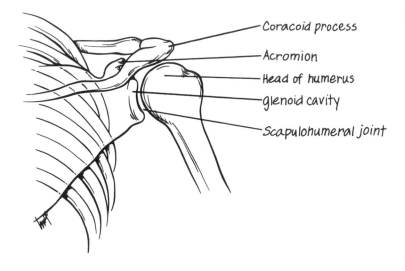

- Coracoid process
- Acromion
- Head of humerus
- glenoid cavity
- Scapulohumeral joint

- The glenohumeral joint can also be demonstrated using a 35 to 45° posterior oblique position (**Grashey method**).

- The bicipital (intertubercular) groove is demonstrated free of superimposition by employing the tangential projection either inferosuperiorly or superoinferiorly.

- A scapular **Y position** is useful for the evaluation of suspected shoulder dislocations. Place the patient in a 60° anterior oblique position with the injured shoulder toward the film.

ACROMIOCLAVICULAR JOINTS

- AP or PA acromioclavicular (AC) joints are ideally imaged upright, bilaterally, and with and without weights.

CLAVICLE

- Include the AC and sternoclavicular (SC) joints when imaging the clavicle.

- Imaging the clavicle in the PA projection offers improved recorded detail compared to the AP projection.

- A 15 to 25° cephalad central ray angle is required for the AP axial clavicle position. The central ray angle is directed 15 to 25° caudad when using the PA axial position.

SCAPULA

- Abduct the arm 90° and direct the central ray to enter 2 in. inferior to the coracoid process when an AP scapula is being imaged.

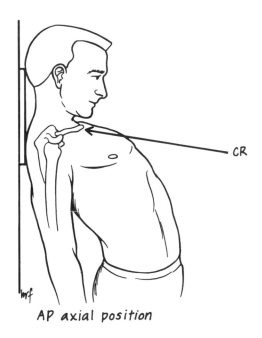

CR

AP axial position

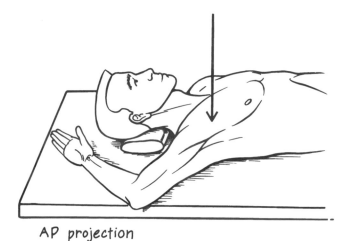

AP projection

- The lateral scapula position is achieved with the patient in a 45 to 60° anterior oblique position, with the affected side toward the film.

- An undesirable increased OID occurs when the lateral scapula is imaged in a posterior oblique position versus an anterior oblique position.

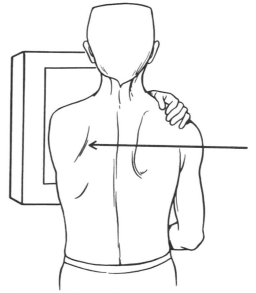

Lateral for body of scapula (≈45° LAO)

Chapter 2 Practice Questions

1. An AP external rotation shoulder position demonstrates the
   a. greater tuberosity.
   b. lesser tuberosity.
   c. AC joints.
   d. glenohumeral joint.

2. A medial oblique elbow position best shows the
   a. radial head.
   b. coranoid process.
   c. coracoid process.
   d. olecranon process.

3. The central ray location for a PA hand projection is the
   a. first PIP joint.
   b. first MP joint.
   c. third MP joint.
   d. second MP joint.

4. The scapular Y shoulder position requires this amount of obliquity.
   a. 30°
   b. 50°
   c. 37°
   d. 60°

5. A PA projection of the hand demonstrates _____ thumb position.
   a. a prone
   b. a lateral
   c. an axial
   d. an oblique

6. Which method is used to demonstrate the glenohumeral joint?
   a. Lawrence
   b. Grashey
   c. Towne
   d. Y

7. Rheumatoid arthritis can be demonstrated with the hands placed in which position?
   a. PA oblique
   b. semiprone
   c. AP oblique
   d. lateral

8. An AP internal rotation shoulder position demonstrates the
   a. coranoid process.
   b. lesser tuberosity.
   c. glenoid fossa.
   d. greater tuberosity.

9. A PA axial clavicle uses a _____ central ray angle.
   a. 10° cephalad
   b. 5° cephalad
   c. 25° caudad
   d. 30° caudad

10. The degree of obliquity necessary for an AP oblique elbow position is
    a. 45°.
    b. 60°.
    c. 30°.
    d. 25°.

11. The hand is _____ for an AP projection of the humerus.
    a. pronated
    b. lateral
    c. supinated
    d. obliqued

12. Which of the following elbow projections best demonstrates the olecranon process?
    a. AP
    b. external oblique
    c. lateral
    d. internal oblique

13. The transthoracic (Lawrence) method helps to demonstrate the
    a. coracoid.
    b. olecranon.
    c. glenohumeral joint.
    d. proximal humerus.

14. The proper centering point for a finger is at the
    a. third MP joint.
    b. PIP joint.
    c. DIP joint.
    d. metacarpal.

15. The humeral epicondyles are _____ to the film when an AP forearm is being imaged.
    a. parallel
    b. perpendicular
    c. rotated
    d. distal

16. AC joints are ideally imaged in which position?

    | 1. supine | a. 1 and 4 |
    | 2. erect | b. 1, 2, and 3 |
    | 3. bilateral | c. 2 and 3 |
    | 4. recumbent | d. all of the above |

17. In imaging the hand, the recommended amount of obliquity is
    a. 15°.
    b. 45°.
    c. 30°.
    d. 60°.

18. An anterior oblique scapula position is preferred over a posterior oblique position because of
    a. simplicity.
    b. the reduced OID.
    c. patient comfort.
    d. the central ray angle.

19. An AP axial clavicle projection requires a _____ central ray angle.
    a. 25° cephalad
    b. 25° caudad
    c. 45° cephalad
    d. 45° caudad

20. Abduct the arm _____ when an AP scapula is being imaged.
    a. 45°.
    b. 60°.
    c. 90°.
    d. 30°.

21. The bicipital (intertubercular) groove is demonstrated using this projection.
    a. PA
    b. lateral
    c. AP
    d. inferosuperior

22. The proper centering point when a thumb is being imaged is at the
    a. MP joint.
    b. PIP joint.
    c. DIP joint.
    d. carpals.

23. A fan lateral hand position effectively separates the
    a. metacarpals.
    b. phalanges.
    c. carpals.
    d. MP joints.

24. Which position is best for the AP oblique ball-catcher projection?
    a. unilateral
    b. 30° oblique
    c. 60° oblique
    d. bilateral

25. The inferosuperior axial position (Lawrence method) demonstrates the
    a. AC joints.
    b. glenohumeral joint.
    c. SC joints.
    d. navicular.

26. For a lateral image the hand is commonly positioned with the _____ aspect against the film.
    a. palmar
    b. radial
    c. ulnar
    d. plantar

27. An AP 45° external oblique elbow projection demonstrates the
    a. radial head.
    b. coracoid process.
    c. coranoid process.
    d. olecranon process.

28. The humeral epicondyles should be _____ to the film when a lateral elbow is being imaged.
    a. AP
    b. parallel
    c. perpendicular
    d. supine

29. Foreign bodies and/or anterior and posterior fracture displacements are demonstrated best when the hand is in which position?

    a. oblique
    b. fan lateral
    c. extension lateral
    d. PA

30. The carpal navicular is undistorted when in which position?

    a. ulnar flexion
    b. radial flexion
    c. semisupine
    d. AP

Lower Extremity

TOES

- The central ray is directed toward the MP joints at an angle of 10 to 15° posteriorly in an AP (dorsoplantar) projection.

- An AP (dorsoplantar) oblique position of the toes requires a 30 to 45° medial rotation.

- Toes are imaged laterally in a lateromedial projection for toes 1 through 3, and in a mediolateral projection for toes 4 and 5. This process reduces the OID.

- The sesamoids near the first MP joint can be imaged using a prone body position with extreme dorsiflexion of the great toe and a tangential central ray direction.

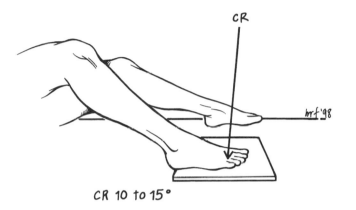

CR 10 to 15°

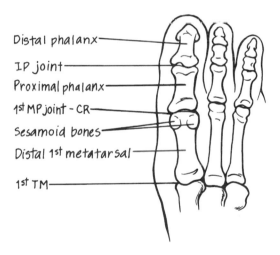

Distal phalanx
IP joint
Proximal phalanx
1st MP joint – CR
Sesamoid bones
Distal 1st metatarsal
1st TM

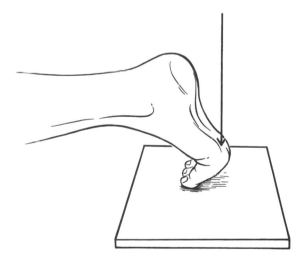

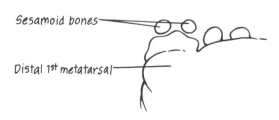

Sesamoid bones
Distal 1st metatarsal

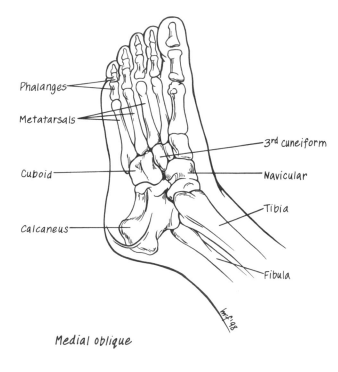

Phalanges

Metatarsals

Cuboid

Calcaneus

3rd cuneiform

Navicular

Tibia

Fibula

Medial oblique

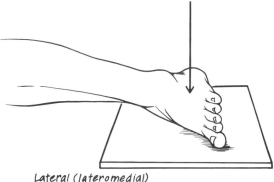

Lateral (lateromedial)

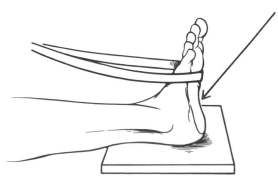

Plantodorsal (axial) projection of calcaneus

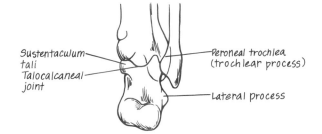

Sustentaculum tali

Talocalcaneal joint

Peroneal trochlea (trochlear process)

Lateral process

FOOT

- In an AP (dorsoplantar) projection of the foot, the central ray is directed 10° posteriorly (toward the heel) in order to better demonstrate the tarsometatarsal joint spaces.

- The central ray location is at the base of the third metatarsal for an AP, oblique, or lateral foot image.

- The foot is rotated medially until the plantar surface forms a 30 to 45° angle to the film when positioning a patient for an oblique foot projection.

- The sinus tarsi, third to fifth metatarsal bases, and most tarsal bones are well visualized using the medial oblique foot position.

- A foot is usually positioned laterally as a mediolateral projection for the sake of patient comfort, however, a lateromedial projection offers a more consistent true lateral image of the foot.

- Weight-bearing (upright) lateral images of the feet can be obtained to demonstrate the structural status of the longitudinal arch.

- The **kite method** for evaluating congenital clubfoot (talipes equinovarus) focuses on the essential need *not* to change the abnormal foot alignment while positioning.

CALCANEUS

- An AP axial calcaneus image requires extreme dorsiflexion of the foot with a 40° cephalad central ray angle entering at the level of the fifth metatarsal base.

ANKLE

- For an AP ankle projection, the foot is dorsiflexed to place the plantar surface perpendicular to the film. The central ray is directed midway between the malleoli.

- For demonstration of the ankle mortise, rotate the leg and foot internally (medially) 15 to 20°. For bony structure evaluation, a 45° medial oblique position is recommended.

- The central ray is directed perpendicular to the ankle at the medial malleolus for a lateral (mediolateral) image.

- Inversion (inward) and eversion (outward) AP stress projections can be employed for the evaluation of ankle joint damage.

LOWER LEG (TIBIA-FIBULA)

- For an AP projection the tibia-fibula is positioned so that the femoral condyles are parallel to the film and the foot is dorsiflexed.

- Flex the knee 45° and ensure that the patella is perpendicular to the cassette when a lateral lower leg is being imaged.

KNEE

- A 5° central ray angle directed toward a point ½ in. inferior to the patellar apex is ideal for the majority of AP knee projections.

- The AP 45° medial (internal) oblique knee position demonstrates the proximal tibio-fibula articulation free of superimposition.

- An optional AP 45° lateral (external) oblique knee position can be used to demonstrate the medial femoral and tibial condyles in profile.

- The 45° PA oblique and AP oblique knee positions demonstrate identical structures. For example, the PA 45° medial oblique position demonstrates proximal tibiofibula articulation, and the PA 45° lateral oblique position demonstrates the medial femoral and tibial condyles in profile.

- Flex the knee 20 to 30° and direct the central ray 5° cephalad to enter 1 in. distal to the medial femoral condyle when the lateral knee is being imaged.

- The intercondylar fossa can be demonstrated by using any one of the following methods
  1. Holmblad (PA axial)
  2. Camp Coventry (PA axial)
  3. Beclere (AP axial).

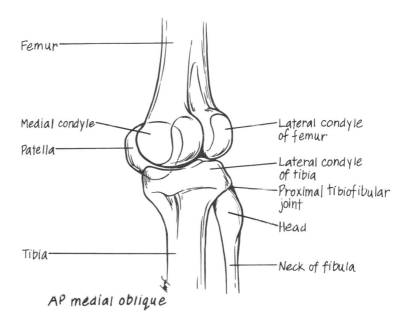

AP medial oblique

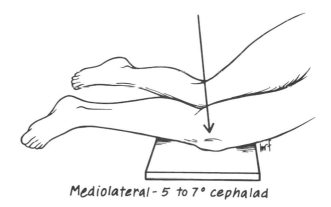

Mediolateral - 5 to 7° cephalad

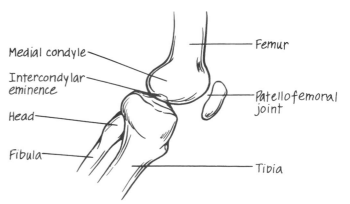

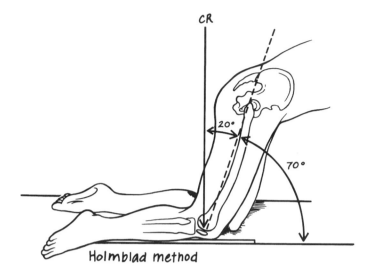

Holmblad method

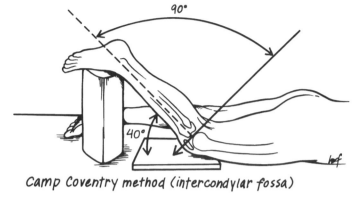

Camp Coventry method (intercondylar fossa)

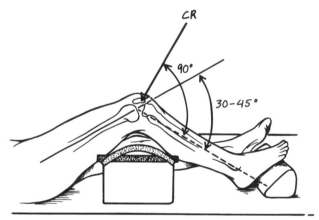

Beclere method

- In the **Holmblad method** the patient is positioned kneeling on the cassette and leaning forward 20 to 30° (approximately 70° knee flexion). Direct the central ray perpendicular to the lower leg centered at the knee joint.

- In the **Camp Coventry method** the patient is prone and the knee is flexed 40 to 50°. Direct the central ray perpendicular to the lower leg centered at the knee joint.

- The **Beclere method** is not preferred because of the increased OID unless a curved cassette is utilized. However, if necessary, position the patient supine with the knee flexed 30 to 45° and direct the central ray in the same fashion as in the previous two positions.

PATELLA

- A lateral patella position demonstrates the patella in profile and patellofemoral articulation and may rule out a transverse fracture. Flex the knee only 5 or 10° so as to prevent further patellar pathology.

- The tangential position found in several methods is useful in ruling out a longitudinal patellar fracture and in demonstrating the patellofemoral articulation.

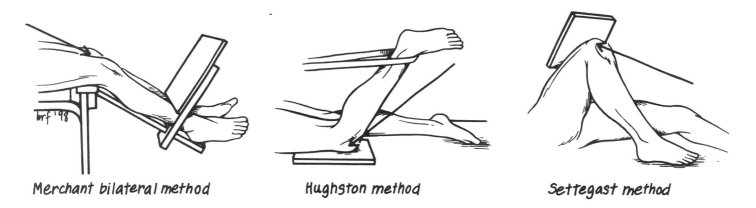

Merchant bilateral method   Hughston method   Settegast method

- Several tangential patella methods are employed, and all require some degree of knee flexion with the central ray angled in such a manner as to properly transit through the patellofemoral articulation. The methods are Merchant bilateral, Hughston, and Settegast (sunrise).

FEMUR

- Internally rotate the toes and lower limb approximately 15° in the imaging of an AP femur in order to demonstrate the proximal femur without foreshortening.

- A true lateral femur projection demonstrates superimposition of the greater and lesser trochanters (proximally) and of the medial and lateral condyles (distally).

PELVIS

- For an AP projection of the pelvis the patient is positioned with both feet internally rotated 15°. The central ray is directed to the (MSP) and 2 in. superior to the pubic symphysis.

- An axial pelvis position (**Chassard-Lapine method**) is useful in demonstrating the relationship between the femoral heads and the acetabula, as well as pelvimetry dimensions.

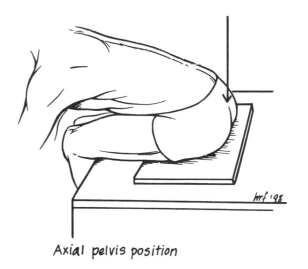

Axial pelvis position

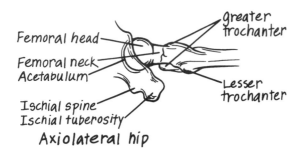

Axiolateral hip

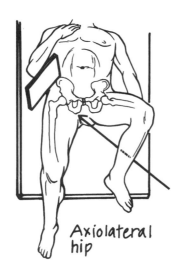

Axiolateral hip

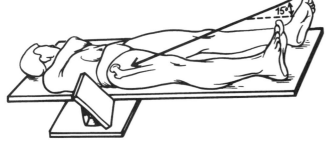

Clements-Nakayama method

HIP

- Internally rotate the foot on the affected side 15° for an AP hip projection in order to overcome anteversion of the femoral neck.

- In a unilateral **frog-leg lateral position** the affected knee is flexed and abducted 40 to 45° from the vertical while the patient is supine.

- A bilateral frog-leg position (modified **Cleaves method**) is used when both hips are to be examined. The patient is supine, with both knees flexed and abducted 40 to 45° from the vertical.

- When leg movement is contraindicated, and a lateral hip image is ordered, any one of several methods can be employed:
    1. Axiolateral position (**Danelius-Miller method**)
    2. Modified axiolateral position (**Clements-Nakayama method**)
    3. Axiolateral position (**Leonard-George method**).

- The methods listed above require practice, experience, and a basic knowledge of femoral neck localizing techniques in order to achieve accuracy and success.

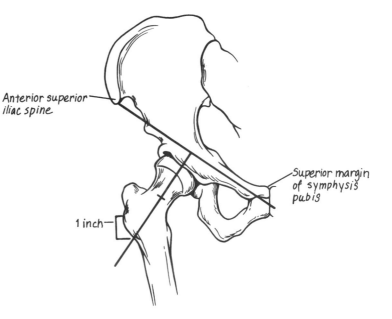

Chapter 3 Practice Questions

1. A foot is positioned obliquely with the plantar surface forming a _____ angle to the film.

   a. 45°
   b. 60°
   c. 10°
   d. 15°

2. The central ray location for an AP knee projection is ½ in. inferior to the patellar _____

   a. base.
   b. ligament.
   c. midline.
   d. apex.

3. An AP projection of the foot requires the central ray to pass through the

   a. third metatarsal head.
   b. third metatarsal base.
   c. third MP joint.
   d. first MP joint.

4. The ankle mortise is demonstrated with a _____ position.

   a. 45° medial oblique
   b. 20° medial oblique
   c. lateral
   d. 45° lateral oblique

5. The central ray angle for an axial calcaneous projection is

   a. 60°.
   b. 45°.
   c. 40°.
   d. 15°.

6. A 45° medial oblique knee projection demonstrates the

   a. patella.
   b. coracoid process.
   c. proximal tibiofibula articulation.
   d. medial condyle.

7. To better demonstrate the tarsometatarsal joint spaces, the central ray is directed

   a. 10° posteriorly.
   b. 10° anteriorly.
   c. 30° caudad.
   d. 45° caudad.

8. A true AP femur image is demonstrated by
   a. a 10° caudad angle.
   b. a 15° toe eversion.
   c. a 15° obliquity.
   d. a 15° toe inversion.

9. The patellar base is found on the _____ surface of the bone.
   a. superior
   b. medial
   c. lateral
   d. inferior

10. The PA axial projection (Camp-Coventry method) is used to demonstrate the
   a. tibiofibula joint.
   b. ankle.
   c. intercondyloid fossa.
   d. patella.

11. A true lateral foot image is obtained more consistently with the _____ sur-face on the film.
   a. plantar
   b. medial
   c. lateral
   d. dorsal

12. Weight-bearing lateral feet projections demonstrate the
   a. longitudinal arch.
   b. mortise joint.
   c. sesamoid bones.
   d. axial arch.

13. For the PA projection (Holmblad method) the patient is positioned with the knee flexed to place the femur angle _____ to the film.
   a. 20°
   b. 70°
   c. 30°
   d. 45°

14. The tangential (Settegast method) projection is used to evaluate the
   a. patella.
   b. hip.
   c. pelvis.
   d. ankle.

15. The central ray location for imaging toes is at the
   a. PIP joints.
   b. metatarsal base.
   c. MP joints.
   d. cuboid.

16. The central ray is directed to enter at the level of the _____ for an AP axial (plantodorsal) calcaneous image.

    a. third MP joint
    b. base of the fifth metatarsal
    c. head of the fifth metatarsal
    d. the fifth MP joint

17. The acetabular dome can be localized by finding the midpoint of a line drawn between the ASIS and the

    a. symphysis pubis.
    b. lesser trochanter.
    c. femoral neck.
    d. femoral head.

18. The kite method is recommended for the evaluation of

    a. Osgood-Schlatter disease.
    b. intercondylar fossae pathology.
    c. talipes equinovarus.
    d. patella fractures.

19. The AP axial position (Beclere method) requires the central ray to be at a right angle to the

    a. patella.
    b. femur.
    c. foot.
    d. lower leg.

20. When lateral toes 1 through 3 are being imaged, the recommended projection is

    a. AP.
    b. lateromedial.
    c. mediolateral.
    d. oblique.

21. The structures best seen with a medial oblique foot position are the

    1. sinus tarsi.
    2. longitudinal arch
    3. intercondylar fossa
    4. third through fifth metatarsal bases.

    a. 1 and 2
    b. 3 and 4
    c. 1 and 4
    d. all of the above

22. The knee is flexed _____ degrees in the lateral position.

    a. 45°
    b. 90°
    c. 40 to 50°
    d. 20 to 30°

23. **The Merchant bilateral method is used to demonstrate**
    a. the patella.
    b. the intercondylar fossa.
    c. club feet.
    d. the ankle mortise.

24. **To demonstrate pelvimetry dimensions the _____ method can be used.**
    a. Settegast
    b. Leonard-George
    c. Holmblad
    d. Chassard-Lapine

25. **In a unilateral frog-leg lateral hip position, the affected leg is abducted _____ degrees from the vertical.**
    a. 60°
    b. 30°
    c. 40°
    d. 25°

26. **An axiolateral position (Danelius-Miller method) is used to image the**
    a. foot.
    b. hip.
    c. knee.
    d. ankle.

27. **The foot should be _____ for an AP ankle projection.**
    a. plantar-flexed
    b. dorsiflexed
    c. everted
    d. inverted

28. **Employ a _____ central ray angle when imaging a lateral knee.**
    a. 30°
    b. 40°
    c. 5°
    d. 90°

29. **Bony structures of the ankle are best shown using this oblique position.**
    a. 15° medial oblique
    b. 45° medial oblique
    c. 15° lateral oblique
    d. 45° lateral oblique

30. **In the Camp-Coventry method the patient is lying in which position?**
    a. supine
    b. oblique
    c. prone
    d. Trendelenburg

Chest and Bony Thorax

- Imaging of the chest is ideal when performed upright (erect) for demonstration of air-fluid levels and also to allow for maximum downward excursion of the diaphragm and to avoid pulmonary vessel engorgement.

- A 72-in. SID is preferred for chest radiography because of the reduction in size distortion (magnification).

- The shoulders are rolled forward when imaging a frontal projection of the chest to remove the scapulae from the lung field.

- The central ray location for a PA chest projection is at the MSP and T7.

- Proper lung aeration is achieved by instructing the patient to take a full inhalation and is evidenced by the visualization of 10 posterior ribs above the diaphragm.

- The heart shadow is demonstrated with less magnification in the PA projection versus the AP projection of the chest.

- A left (versus right) lateral chest position is the position of choice because of the decreased OID of the heart.

- Either PA or AP 45° oblique positions of the chest can be used. PA oblique positions include RAO and LAO which demonstrate the lung field of the up side. AP oblique positions include RPO and LPO which demonstrate the lung field of the down side.

- An AP lordotic projection of the chest demonstrates the lung apices free of clavicular superimposition.

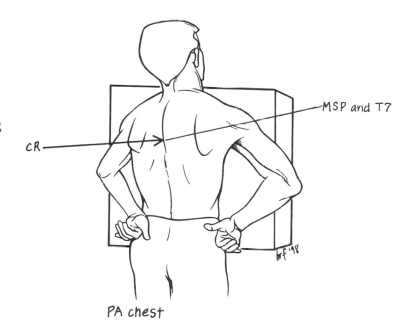

PA chest

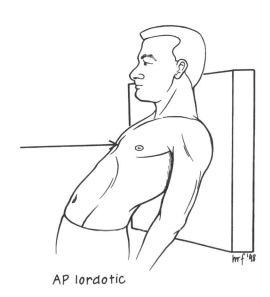

AP lordotic

- A central ray angle of 15 to 20° cephalad can be used when the patient cannot be positioned in the lordotic fashion.

- Decubitus positions of the chest generally demonstrate "fluid down" or "free air up."

- In the lateral decubitus position the patient is lying on the affected side, in the ventral decubitus position the patient is prone, and in the dorsal decubitus position the patient is supine. The central ray orientation for *all* decubitus positions is directed horizontally.

STERNUM

- A 15 to 20° RAO position projects the sternum into the homogeneous heart shadow.

- The patient is instructed to take shallow breaths during the RAO sternum exposure in order to blur the pulmonary markings.

- An optimum 60 to 72-in. SID is recommended for a lateral sternum projection to reduce sternal magnification caused by the increased OID.

- The lateral sternum is imaged with sharper detail when the patient is erect and has the arms drawn back and respiration is suspended at the end of deep inspiration.

STERNOCLAVICULAR JOINTS

- When imaging the SC joints in a PA projection, direct the central ray perpendicular to T3.

- PA oblique positions (RAO and LAO) with a 15 to 20° rotation best demonstrate the downside SC joint.

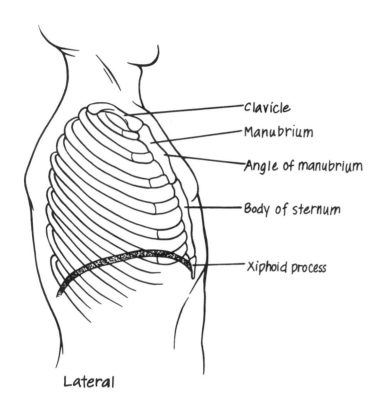

Clavicle
Manubrium
Angle of manubrium
Body of sternum
Xiphoid process

Lateral

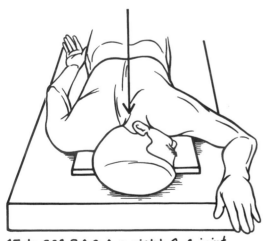

15 to 20° RAO for right S-C joints

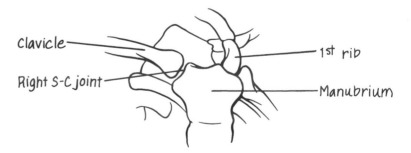

Clavicle
Right S-C joint
1st rib
Manubrium

RIBS

- The upper ribs are best imaged when the patient is erect on inspiration, and the lower ribs are best demonstrated when the patient is supine on expiration.

- PA rib projections best show anterior rib injuries, whereas AP projections best show posterior rib injuries.

- An erect PA chest projection is commonly included with rib imaging protocol to rule out respiratory pathology such as pneumothorax or hemothorax.

- The downside axillary rib portion is demonstrated with a 45° RPO or LPO (AP oblique) position.

- The 45° RAO or LAO (PA oblique) position is utilized to demonstrate the upside axillary rib portion.

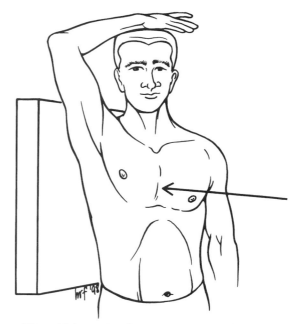

RPO (injury to the right posterior ribs above diaphragm

Chapter 4 Practice Questions

1. An AP lordotic projection of the chest best demonstrates
   a. air-fluid levels.
   b. the sternum.
   c. lung apices.
   d. the diaphragm.

2. Proper lung aeration is evidenced when _____ posterior ribs are seen above the diaphragm.
   a. 8
   b. 10
   c. 12
   d. 7

3. The RPO position of the lungs best demonstrates the _____ lung field.
   a. left
   b. right
   c. lower
   d. upper

4. For a frontal projection of the chest, a PA position is preferred because it demonstrates
   a. air-fluid levels.
   b. reduced heart magnification.
   c. apical superimposition.
   d. less motion.

5. The amount of obliquity used in chest radiography is
   a. 45°.
   b. 60°.
   c. 30°.
   d. 10°.

6. Ideal breathing for chest imaging is
   a. quiet breathing.
   b. noisy breathing.
   c. full exhalation.
   d. full inhalation.

7. Rolling the shoulders forward for frontal chest images helps to remove the
   _____ from the lung fields.
   a. scapulae
   b. arms
   c. clavicles
   d. AC joints

8. Why is a 72-in. SID preferred for chest radiography?
   a. patient comfort
   b. air-fluid levels
   c. heart magnification
   d. motion

9. The central ray location for a PA chest projection is at the level of
   a. C7.
   b. T5.
   c. T7.
   d. L3.

10. The oblique sternum is best visualized using which position?
    a. 15 to 20° LAO
    b. 15 to 20° RAO
    c. 45° RAO
    d. 45° LAO

11. The upper ribs are best imaged in which position?
    a. upright
    b. supine
    c. recumbent
    d. decubitus

12. AP rib projections best demonstrate the _____ ribs.
    a. lower
    b. upper
    c. anterior
    d. posterior

13. Why is a left lateral chest projection preferred over a right lateral chest projection?

    a. reduced heart motion
    b. reduced heart magnification
    c. increased heart OID
    d. patient comfort

14. A left lateral decubitus chest projection utilizes a _____ central ray.

    a. 30° angle
    b. parallel
    c. vertical
    d. horizontal

15. The RAO sternum position demonstrates the sternum within the

    a. diaphragm.
    b. clavicles.
    c. heart shadow.
    d. T-spine.

16. The central ray location for SC joints is at the level of

    a. T7.
    b. T3.
    c. C7.
    d. T5.

17. An erect PA chest projection is usually included in routine rib imaging protocol in order to rule out

    a. rib fractures.
    b. clavicle displacement.
    c. pneumothorax.
    d. sternal separation.

18. A RPO SC joint image demonstrates which of the _____ SC joints open?

    a. left
    b. right
    c. both
    d. neither

19. An AP oblique rib position best shows the

    a. downside axillary.
    b. upper posterior.
    c. upside axillary.
    d. lower anterior.

20. Posterior oblique rib positions best demonstrate the _____ ribs.

    a. upper posterior
    b. downside axillary
    c. lower anterior
    d. upside axillary

Abdomen

- An AP (supine) projection of the abdomen is often referred to as a **KUB** (kidneys, ureters, and bladder).

- The central ray location for a KUB is at the MSP and the IC.

- An AP upright abdomen or left lateral decubitus film demonstrates air-fluid levels and/or accumulations of gas or free intra-abdominal air. The central ray and film centering must be high enough to include the diaphragm.

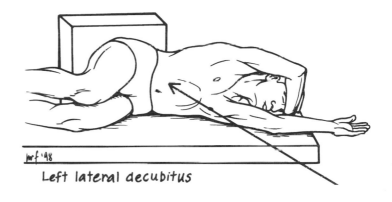

Left lateral decubitus

- Both the upright abdomen and left lateral decubitus positions require a horizontal central ray. Be careful to wait a minimum of 5 min. after positioning before taking the exposure (to allow the air and fluid to settle naturally).

- A left or right dorsal decubitus position of the abdomen can be used to demonstrate aneurysms, vascular calcifications, or air-fluid levels.

- The term **acute abdominal series (AAS)** refers to three images taken for a protocol in sequence:
  1. AP supine abdomen
  2. Erect (upright or lateral decubitus) abdomen
  3. PA chest

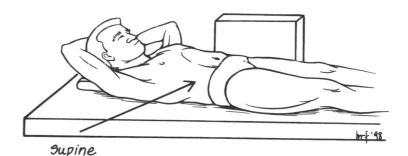

Supine

Chapter 5 Practice Questions

1. A decubitus position requires the use of a _____ central ray.

   a. vertical
   b. horizontal
   c. axial
   d. tangential

2. An AP (supine) projection of the abdomen is often called a

   a. KGB.
   b. KBU.
   c. KUB.
   d. AAS.

3. A dorsal decubitus position is most similar to

   a. prone.
   b. oblique.
   c. lateral.
   d. supine.

4. A position alternative to the upright abdomen position is

   a. KUB.
   b. prone.
   c. left lateral decubitus.
   d. right lateral decubitus.

5. The central ray location for a KUB is at the

   a. MSP and the IC.
   b. MCP and the IC.
   c. MSP and the ASIS.
   d. MCP and the ASIS.

6. Free fluid accumulates on the patient's _____ in a dorsal decubitus position.

   a. anterior surface
   b. posterior surface
   c. left side
   d. right side

7. An AP erect abdomen image must include the

   a. pubic bone.
   b. diaphragm.
   c. tenth rib.
   d. heart shadow.

8. An acute abdominal series consists of _____ positions.

   a. two
   b. four
   c. three
   d. five

9. Allow a minimum of _____ min. for fluid or air to settle when imaging with a horizontal central ray.

   a. 5
   b. 10
   c. 15
   d. 20

10. Which position is most often used to demonstrate an aneurysm?

    a. ventral decubitus
    b. dorsal decubitus
    c. erect
    d. KUB

Vertebral Column

CHAPTER 6

CERVICAL SPINE

- Cervical vertebra 1 is referred to as the **atlas**, and cervical vertebra 2 is called the **axis**.

- C1 and C2 are ideally imaged through the AP **open mouth projection.** This position is achieved when, with the mouth wide open, the head is adjusted so that an imaginary line from the lower edge (occlusal plane) of the upper incisors to the mastoid tips is perpendicular to the film.

- The **dens (odontoid process)** is a structure that forms the most superior portion of C2 (the axis).

- To correct a poorly positioned open mouth AP projection, determine which structure is superimposed on the dens. When the upper teeth are superimposed on the dens, increase the degree of neck extension; if the occipital bone is superimposed on the dens, increase the degree of neck flexion.

- If the upper dens cannot be demonstrated with an open mouth position, the Fuchs or the Judd method can be used.

- The **Fuchs method** involves an AP projection with the chin extended, demonstrating the dens within the foramen magnum.

- The **Judd method** is a PA projection of the dens (as seen through the foramen magnum), with the orbitomeatal line (OML) positioned 37° to the plane of the film.

- An AP axial cervical spine (C-spine) projection utilizes a 15 to 20° cephalad central ray angle to better reveal the intervertebral disk spaces.

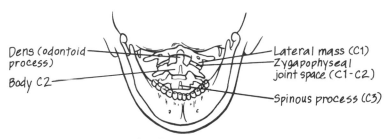

Dens (odontoid process)
Body C2
Lateral mass (C1)
Zygapophyseal joint space (C1-C2)
Spinous process (C3)

AP open mouth, C1-C2

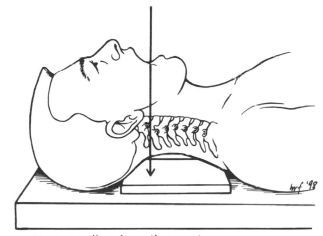

Open mouth spine alignment

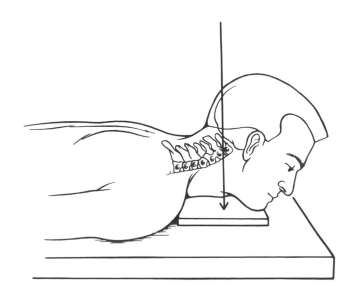

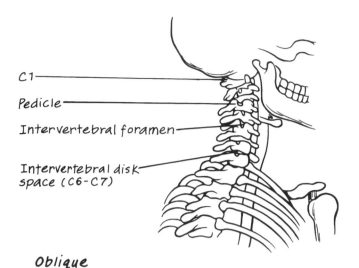

C1
Pedicle
Intervertebral foramen
Intervertebral disk space (C6-C7)

Oblique

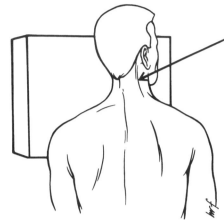

Erect LAO position. CR 15 to 20° caudad (less thyroid exposure).

- PA oblique projections (RAO or LAO) of the C-spine demonstrate the downside (closest to the film) intervertebral foramina. The patient is rotated 45°, and a central ray angle of 15 to 20° caudad is used. (Rule: the patient is face down, side down, and angle down.)

- AP oblique projections (RPO or LPO) of the C-spine demonstrate the upside (farthest from the film) intervertebral foramina. The patient is rotated 45°, and a central ray angle of 15 to 20° cephalad is used. (Rule: the patient is face up, side up, and angle up.)

- A true lateral C-spine image demonstrates all seven cervical bodies, intervertebral joint spaces, spinous processes, and zygapophyseal joints.

- The use of a 72-in. SID helps to compensate for the increase in OID and is recommended for both lateral and oblique C-spine images.

- Lateral flexion and extension C-spine images help to demonstrate range of motion as affected by trauma or disease.

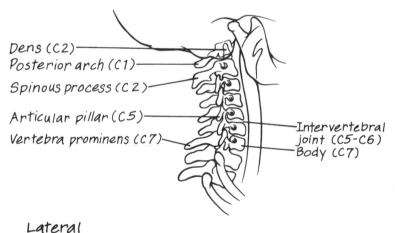

Dens (C2)
Posterior arch (C1)
Spinous process (C2)
Articular pillar (C5)
Vertebra prominens (C7)
Intervertebral joint (C5-C6)
Body (C7)

Lateral

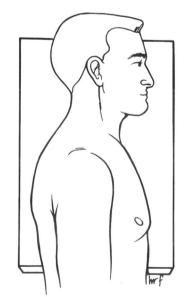

Erect L lateral (front to back centering).

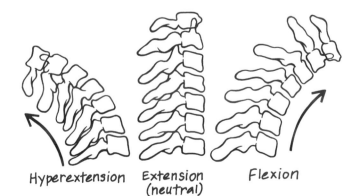

Hyperextension   Extension (neutral)   Flexion

- It may be necessary to place a "thick-shouldered" patient in a **swimmer's lateral position** in order to visualize the lower cervical and uppermost thoracic region.

- The upright (erect) swimmer's lateral position is called the **Twining method**.

- The recumbent swimmer's lateral position is known as the **Pawlow method**.

- Both these methods require elevation (raising) of the dependent arm and depression (lowering) of the nondependent arm, which effectively separate the thick shoulder region.

- A C-spine vertebral arch position (an AP axial projection) utilizes a 20 to 30° caudad central ray angle directed to exit at C7.

- An AP **chewing** or **wagging jaw projection (Ottonello method)** provides an AP image of the entire C-spine with a blurred mandible.

THORACIC SPINE

- The central ray location for an AP T-spine projection is at T7.

- In the lateral T-spine position the median coronal plane is perpendicular to the film, demonstrating the vertebral bodies, intervertebral joint spaces, and intervertebral foramina.

- The 70° posterior oblique (RPO and LPO) positions demonstrate the upside zygapophyseal joints, whereas the anterior oblique (RAO and LAO) positions demonstrate the downside joints.

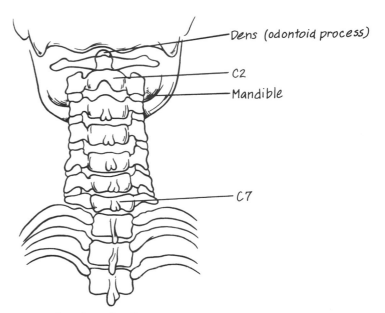

AP "chewing"

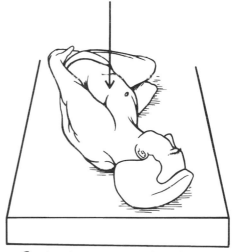

Posterior oblique (RPO)

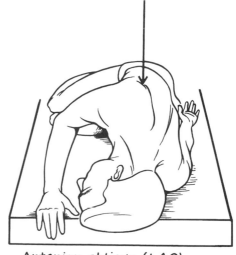

Anterior oblique (LAO)

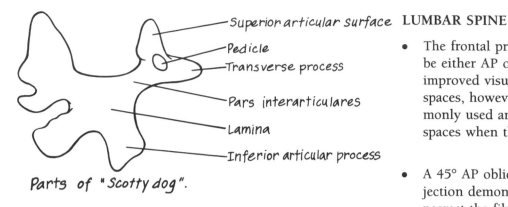

Parts of "Scotty dog".

- Superior articular surface
- Pedicle
- Transverse process
- Pars interarticulares
- Lamina
- Inferior articular process

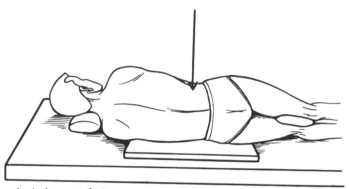

L lateral (CR perpendicular to film).

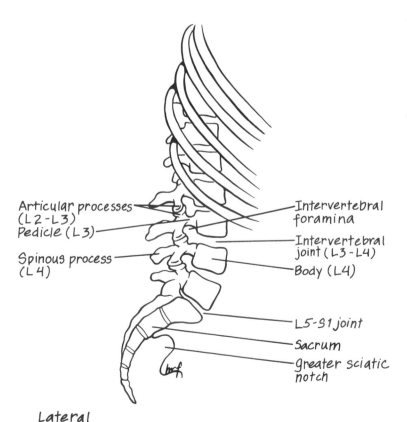

- Articular processes (L2-L3)
- Pedicle (L3)
- Spinous process (L4)
- Intervertebral foramina
- Intervertebral joint (L3-L4)
- Body (L4)
- L5-S1 joint
- Sacrum
- Greater sciatic notch

Lateral

LUMBAR SPINE

- The frontal projection of the lumbar spine can be either AP or PA. The PA projection offers improved visualization of the intervertebral spaces, however, the AP projection is commonly used and can demonstrate open interspaces when the knees and hips are flexed.

- A 45° AP oblique (RPO or LPO) L-spine projection demonstrates the zygapophyseal joints nearest the film.

- 45° AP oblique (RAO and LAO) projections of the L-spine demonstrate the upside zygapophyseal joints.

- The oblique position and the resultant film are considered successful when the "Scottie dog sign" is visualized. The Scottie image is formed by different structures of vertebrae.

- A lateral lumbar spine position may require a caudal central ray angle when the spine is *not* adjusted parallel to the film.

- The central ray angle for a lateral lumbar spine and/or a L5 to S1 position (lumbosacral junction) varies. The angle is 5° caudad for a male and 8° caudad for a female.

- The condition of scoliosis can be evaluated when imaging the thoracic and lumbar spine together on a 14 × 17 lengthwise film. Two AP or PA exposures are taken, one erect and one recumbent, for comparison.

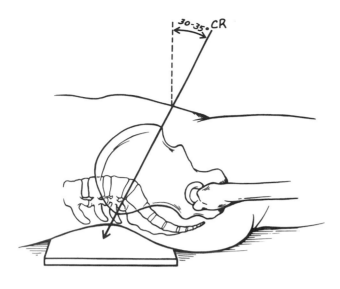

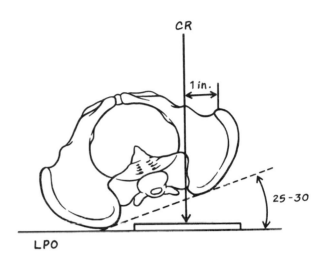

LPO

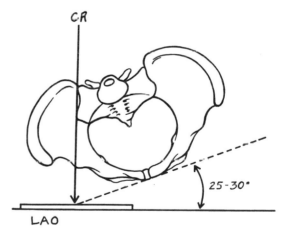

LAO

SACROILIAC JOINTS

- An AP axial sacroiliac (SI) joint image requires a central ray angle of 30 to 35° cephalad to enter the MSP at the level of the ASIS. For PA projection use a caudad central ray angle.

- SI joints are demonstrated open when the patient is obliqued 25 to 30°. The AP oblique (RPO or LPO) position opens the upside SI joint, and the PA oblique position (RAO or LAO) opens the downside.

SACRUM

- An AP axial sacrum projection uses a 15° cephalad angle directed at the MSP and halfway between the ASIS and the symphysis pubis.

- When the patient is prone for sacrum imaging, angle the central ray 15° caudad.

- Separate AP projections of the sacrum and coccyx are required, however, the lateral image can include both if centered properly.

COCCYX

- An AP axial coccyx projection uses a 10° caudad central ray angle, whereas the PA axial projection requires a 10° cephalad angle.

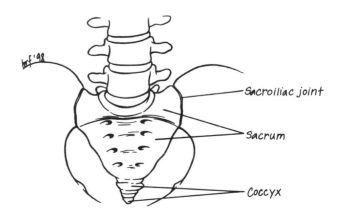

1. The PA projection of the dens (Judd method) is positioned with the OML _____ to the film.
   a. 30°
   b. 37°
   c. 45°
   d. 90°

2. The _____ position or projection best demonstrates the joint space between the inferior and superior articulating processes.
   a. AP
   b. AP oblique
   c. lateral
   d. PA oblique

3. The Scottie dog sign is seen when the _____ is being imaged.
   a. T-spine
   b. sacrum
   c. C-spine
   d. L-spine

4. A RAO C-spine position demonstrates the
   a. right zygapophyseal joints.
   b. left intervertebral foramina.
   c. right intervertebral foramina.
   d. left zygapophyseal joints.

5. A lateral lumbar spine position for a female patient may require a _____ central ray angle.
   a. 5° cephalad
   b. 5° caudad
   c. 8° caudad
   d. 15° caudad

6. Which projection of the lumbar spine offers improved visualization of the disk spaces?
   a. PA
   b. AP
   c. AP axial
   d. PA axial

7. The central ray angle and direction for an AP C-spine projection is
   a. 45° cephalad.
   b. 15 to 20° cephalad.
   c. 45° caudad.
   d. 15 to 20° caudad.

8. The wagging jaw (Ottonello method) projection is used to demonstrate
   a. the C7/T1 junction.
   b. C1 and C2.
   c. the oblique C-spine.
   d. the entire AP C-spine.

9. Oblique C-spine positions require the patient to be rotated
   a. 15°.
   b. 20°.
   c. 35°.
   d. 45°.

10. The Fuchs method is used to demonstrate
    a. the odontoid process.
    b. C7.
    c. chin flexion.
    d. the intervertebral foramina.

11. The right zygapophyseal joints are visualized when the T-spine is in which position?
    a. lateral
    b. AP
    c. 70° LPO
    d. 70° RPO

12. To better visualize the intervertebral spaces in a PA C-spine projection, direct the central ray
    a. 45° to the feet.
    b. 15° to the head.
    c. 15° to the feet.
    d. 45° to the head.

13. An AP open mouth projection of the dens results in a radiograph with the occipital bone superimposed on the dens. What corrective action should be taken?
    a. Use an angle 20° caudad.
    b. None.
    c. Raise the chin.
    d. Tuck in the chin.

14. The central ray location for an AP T-spine projection is at
    a. T3.
    b. T7.
    c. C7.
    d. T5.

15. The amount of patient rotation necessary to best visualize open SI joints is
    a. 10°.
    b. 15°.
    c. 25°.
    d. 45°.

16. A right PA oblique position of the lumbar spine best demonstrates the
    a. left zygapophyseal joint.
    b. right zygapophyseal joint.
    c. left intervertebral foramina.
    d. right intervertebral foramina.

17. For imaging the coccyx, the central ray is angled _____ when the patient is in the prone position.
    a. 10° cephalad
    b. 15° cephalad
    c. 10° caudad
    d. 15° caudad

18. Cervical vertebra 2 is referred to as the
    a. vertebra prominens.
    b. atlas.
    c. dens.
    d. axis.

19. A PA axial sacral image requires a _____ central ray angle.
    a. 10° caudad
    b. 15° caudad
    c. 10° cephalad
    d. 15° cephalad

20. A 25° RAO position opens up the _____ SI joints.
    a. upside
    b. left
    c. right
    d. middle

21. The dens is located on the superior aspect of
    a. C1.
    b. C2.
    c. C7.
    d. C5.

22. Range of motion in the neck can be evaluated with this position.
    a. PA oblique
    b. PA axial
    c. lateral flexion or extension
    d. AP axial

23. The midcoronal plane is _____ to the film in the lateral T-spine position.
    a. parallel
    b. perpendicular
    c. lateral
    d. oblique

24. An upright swimmer's lateral position is known as the _____ method.

    a. Twining
    b. Fuchs
    c. Judd
    d. Pawlow

25. A 45° LPO lumbar spine position demonstrates the _____ zygapophyseal joints.

    a. right
    b. bilateral
    c. upside
    d. left

26. The condition of scoliosis can be evaluated by imaging the

    a. dens.
    b. T- and L-spine.
    c. C-spine.
    d. sacrum.

27. In order to image the downside SI joints the patient is in which position?

    a. RAO or LPO
    b. RPO or LAO
    c. RAO or LAO
    d. RPO or LPO

28. C1 is given the name

    a. atlas.
    b. axis.
    c. dens.
    d. odontoid.

29. An imaginary line from the occlusal plane of the upper incisors to the _____ is perpendicular to the film when the patient is positioned for the open mouth projection.

    a. odontoid
    b. external auditory meatus
    c. mastoids
    d. mentum

30. In the swimmer's lateral position, the patient's dependent arm is

    a. raised.
    b. lowered.
    c. forward.
    d. adducted.

Head Work

SURFACE LANDMARKS AND POSITIONING LINES

- The **superciliary ridge (arch)** is a ridge of bone above each eye extending across the forehead.

- There is a slight depression above the superciliary ridge termed the **supraorbital groove**.

- The **glabella** is a smooth, depressed area between and slightly above the eyebrows.

- The depression at the junction of the nasal bones and frontal bone (the bridge of the nose) is termed the **nasion**.

- The **acanthion** is a midline point where the nasal septum and upper lip meet.

- The angle of the mandible is termed the **gonion**.

- The anterior portion of the chin (the mentum) is called the **mental point**.

- The opening of the external ear canal is called the **external auditory meatus (EAM)**.

- The area where the top of the ear forms an attachment to the head is termed the **top of ear attachment (TEA)**.

- The inner junction of the eyelids is called the **inner canthus**, and the outer junction is called the **outer canthus**.

- The upper rim of the orbit is termed the **supraorbital margin (SOM)**, and the lower rim is called the **infraorbital margin (IOM)**.

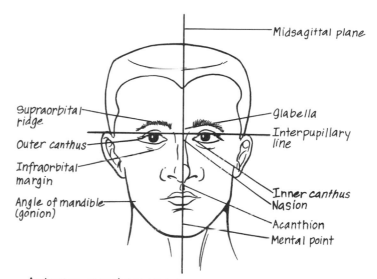

Anterior aspect landmarks.

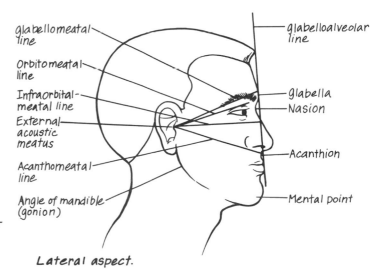

Lateral aspect.

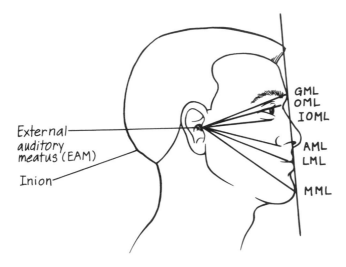

GML = glabellomeatal line
OML = Orbitomeatal line
IOML = Infraorbitomeatal line
AML = Acanthiomeatal line
LML = Lipsmeatal line
MML = Mentomeatal line

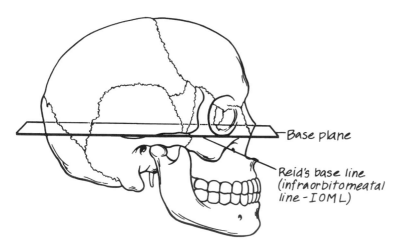

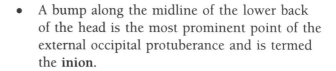

- A bump along the midline of the lower back of the head is the most prominent point of the external occipital protuberance and is termed the **inion**.

- An imaginary line between the eyes is known as the **interpupillary line (IPL)**.

- The **glabellomeatal line (GML)** is a line from the glabella to the EAM.

- The most common positioning line used for head work is the **orbitomeatal line (OML)**, which runs from the outer canthus to the EAM.

- The **infraorbitomeatal line (IOML)** connects the infraorbital margin to the EAM and is often referred to as **Reid's baseline**.

- There is a 7° difference between the OML and the IOML, and an 8° difference between the GML and the OML. Knowing these differences helps the radiographer to make central ray angle adjustments when positioning the patient.

- The **acanthiomeatal line (AML)** is a line connecting the acanthion and the EAM.

- A line running from the mental point to the EAM is called the **mentomeatal line (MML)**.

- In patients positioned for the imaging of tangential nasal bones, the **glabelloalveolar line (GAL)** is used. This line connects the glabella to an anterior point of the alveolar processes of the maxilla.

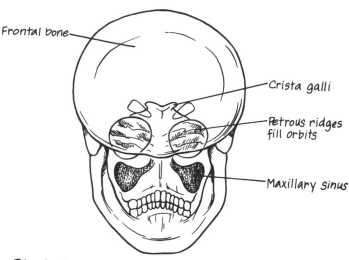

Frontal bone

Crista galli

Petrous ridges
fill orbits

Maxillary sinus

PA skull

SKULL

- A PA skull projection without a central ray angle demonstrates the petrous pyramids filling the orbits and is the primary projection for imaging the frontal bone.

- The PA axial projection (**Caldwell method**) requires a 15° caudad central ray angle to exit the nasion.

- Both the PA and PA axial projections are positioned with the MSP and OML perpendicular to the film.

- The AP axial projection (**Towne method**) utilizes a 30° caudad central ray angle when the chin is tucked in enough to place the OML perpendicular to the film.

- If the patient's chin cannot be tucked in enough, direct the central ray 37°to the IOML.

- There is a 7° difference between the OML and the IOML.

- The PA **Haas method** is an alternative to the AP Towne method, using a 25° cephalad central ray angle.

- Both the PA Haas and AP Towne methods demonstrate the occipital region of the cranium.

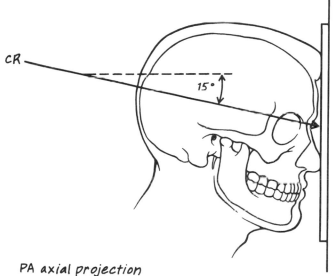

CR

15°

PA axial projection

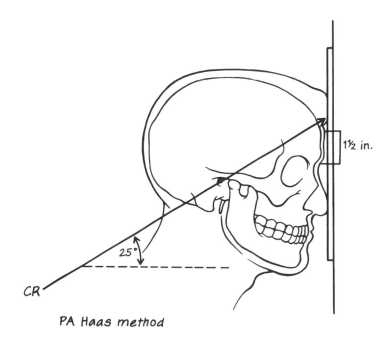

1½ in.

25°

CR

PA Haas method

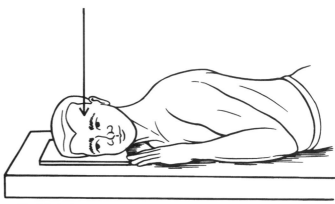

Right lateral

- The lateral skull position places the head in a true lateral position with the MSP parallel and the IPL perpendicular to the film.

- The base of the skull can be imaged using the submentovertical (SMV) (full basal, Schuller method) projection.

- For the SMV projection, the patient is positioned with the IOML parallel to the film, and the central ray is directed perpendicular to the IOML midway between the mandibular angles.

- The reverse of the SMV projection is the verticosubmental projection, requiring the central ray to enter the vertex of the skull and exit the base.

- An alternative method for imaging the skull base is the **Lysholm method.** Place the head in a true lateral position using a 35° caudad angle that exits 1 in. distal to the EAM.

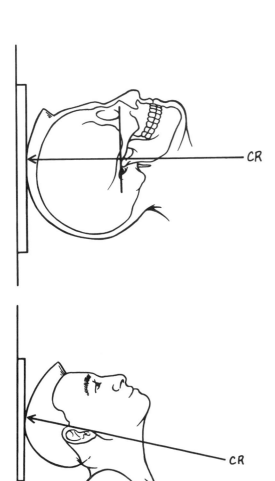

Submentovertex

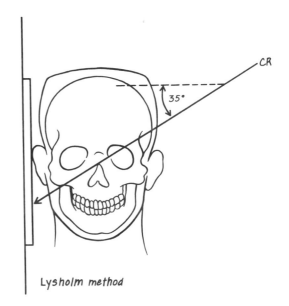

Lysholm method

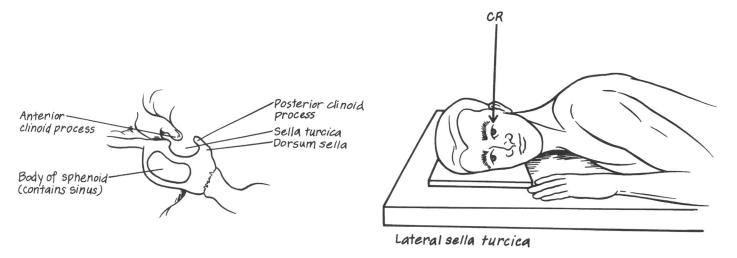

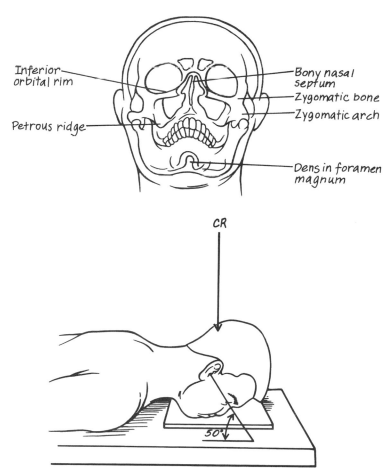

Lateral sella turcica

SELLA TURCICA

- A lateral projection requires the central ray to be aligned perpendicular to a point ¾ in. anterior and ¾ in. superior to the EAM.

- An AP projection of the sella is achieved using the Towne method (30 to 37° caudad central ray angle).

- A PA projection of the sella requires use of the Haas method (25° cephalad central ray angle).

FACIAL BONES

- Imaging of the lateral facial bones requires a true lateral head position (MSP parallel and IPL perpendicular to the film) with the central ray aimed at the zygoma.

- The parietoacanthial projection (**Waters method**) employs a PA position with the MML perpendicular to the film, which places the OML 37° to the film.

- When correctly performed, the Waters method demonstrates the petrous ridges just below the maxillary sinuses.

- For a modified Waters method the patient is positioned with the OML 55° to the plane of the film. This position best shows the floor of the orbits.

- The central ray exits the acanthion for both the parietoacanthial projection (Waters method) and the modified Waters method.

- The reverse Waters method is called the **acanthoparietal projection.**

Modified parietoacanthia (Waters)- Recumbent.
-LML perpendicular (OML)

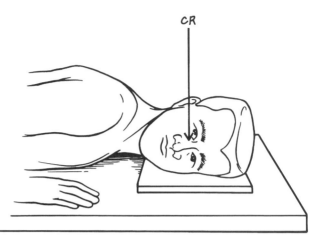

Left lateral

NASAL BONES

- The right and left lateral nasal bones are generally examined for comparison.

- The central ray location for the lateral nasal bones is ½ to ¾ in. distal to the nasion.

- The superoinferior (tangential) projection requires the central ray to be parallel to the GAL.

ZYGOMATIC ARCHES

- An SMV projection demonstrates the bilateral zygomatic arches. Be careful to align the IOML parallel to the film.

- From the position for the SMV projection, rotate the MSP and tilt the chin 15° toward the side of interest to achieve a tangential (oblique) projection of one zygomatic arch.

- The AP axial projection (Towne method) is useful for imaging zygomatic arches when the central ray location is adjusted to enter the glabella.

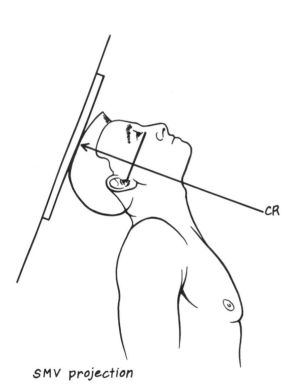

SMV projection

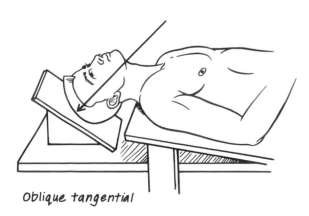

Oblique tangential

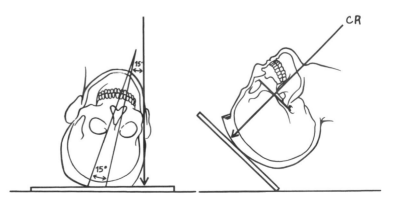

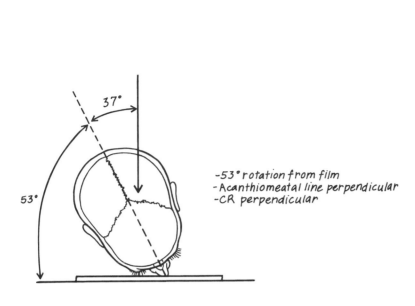

37°

53°

-53° rotation from film
-Acanthiomeatal line perpendicular
-CR perpendicular

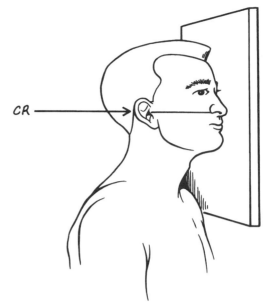

CR

Parieto-orbital projection

OPTIC FORAMINA (ORBITS)

- The optic foramina are imaged bilaterally for comparison.

- For the parietoorbital projection (PA **Rhese method**), the patient's head rests on the chin, cheek, and nose. Adjust the AML perpendicular to the film and place the MSP 53° to the film.

- The PA Rhese method demonstrates the downside orbit.

- An orbitoparietal projection (AP Rhese method) demonstrates the upside orbit and is not preferred because of the magnification caused by the increased OID.

- When positioned properly, the optic foramen can be visualized in the lower outer quadrant of the orbital shadow.

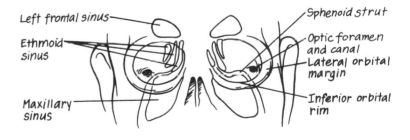

Left frontal sinus

Ethmoid sinus

Maxillary sinus

Sphenoid strut

Optic foramen and canal

Lateral orbital margin

Inferior orbital rim

MANDIBLE

- A PA mandible projection without a central ray angle best demonstrates the rami and the lateral portion of the mandibular body.

- A PA 20 to 25° cephalad axial projection with the OML and the MSP perpendicular to the film demonstrates the condylar processes.

- An axiolateral projection using a 25° cephalad angle images the ramus well.

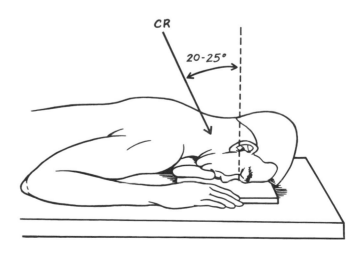

CR

20-25°

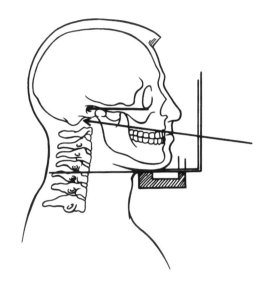

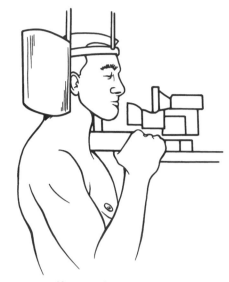

Orthopan tomogram

- From the lateral oblique position rotate the mandible 30° toward the film for demonstration of the body, or 45° for the mentum, while still using a 25° cephalad central ray angle.

- A panorex (orthopantomogram) demonstrates the entire mandible (including the TMJs) in a panoramic fashion.

TEMPOROMANDIBULAR JOINTS

- Bilateral open and closed mouth positions may be required for all images of the TMJs for comparison purposes.

- An AP 35° caudad axial projection (modified Towne method) can be used with the central ray centered at the TMJs and the MSP.

- The axiolateral (transcranial) projection (**Schuller method**) requires a true lateral head position and a central ray direction of 25 to 30° caudad.

- For a lateral transfacial projection (**Albers-Schonberg method**) the patient is positioned with the head in a true lateral position using a 20° cephalad central ray angle.

- The **Pirie method** (axial transoral position) demonstrates the sphenoidal sinuses through an open mouth.

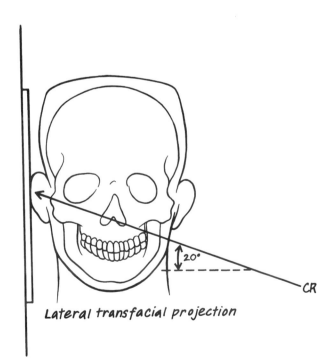

Lateral transfacial projection

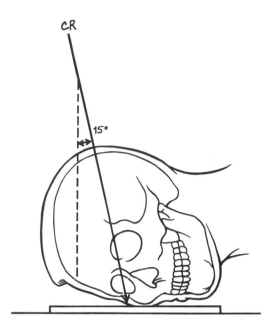

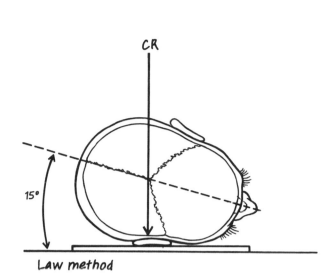

Law method

MASTOIDS

- Both mastoids are usually imaged for comparison.

- When using the **Law method** (axiolateral oblique projection), the central ray is directed to enter 1 to 2 in. posterior and superior to the upside EAM.

- The Law method involves a 15° oblique face position with a 15° caudad central ray angle.

- The Law method demonstrates a lateral perspective of the mastoid cells closest to the film.

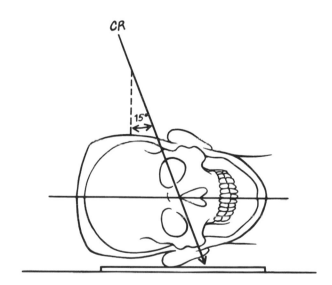

MASTOID AND PETROUS PORTIONS

- Axiolateral positions include the
    1. **Henschen method**, 15° caudad angle
    2. **Schuller method**, 25° caudad angle
    3. **Lysholm method**, 35° caudad angle.

- The AP axial projection (Towne method) demonstrates the petrous ridges above the base of the skull.

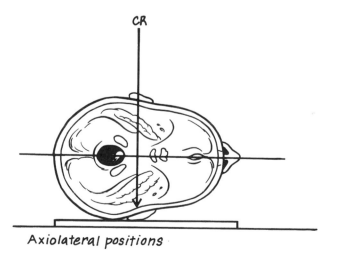

Axiolateral positions

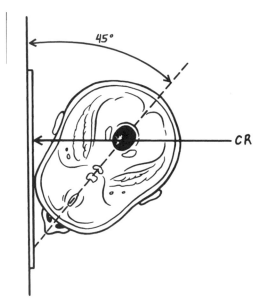

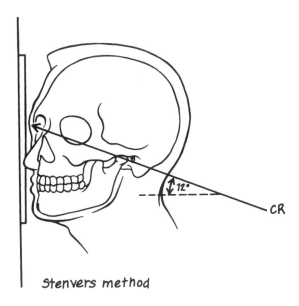

Stenvers method

- The **Stenvers method** (axiolateral oblique or posterior profile) requires a position with the head rotated 45° (from the PA position) toward the side of interest, the IOML perpendicular to the film, and a 12° cephalad central ray angle.

- The Stenvers method demonstrates the downside petrous bone in profile and the downside mastoid.

- The reverse of the Stenvers method is the **Arcelin method** (anterior profile projection), which utilizes a 10° caudad angle and demonstrates the upside petrous bone and mastoid.

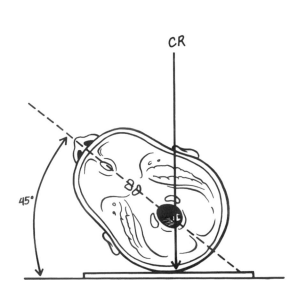

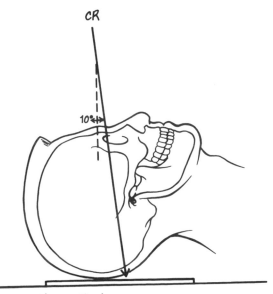

Arcelin method

- The **Mayer method** (axioposterior oblique) requires a 45° head rotation (from the AP position) toward the side of interest and the central ray angled 45° caudad centered through the downside EAM.

- The **Owen** (modified Mayer's) **method** involves only a 30 to 40° head rotation with only a 30 to 40° caudad central ray angle.

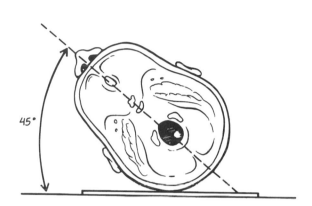

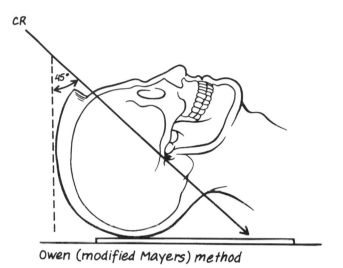

Owen (modified Mayers) method

Chapter 7 Practice Questions

1. A lateral transcranial projection demonstrates the
   a. sella turcica.
   b. frontal sinus.
   c. TMJs.
   d. sphenoid sinus.

2. This structure is seen below the maxillary sinuses in the parietoacanthial projection.
   a. nasal septum
   b. petrous ridges
   c. sella turcica
   d. orbits

3. When rotating the head as in the Rhese method, the principal structure of interest is the
   a. optic foramen.
   b. skull base.
   c. zygomatic arch.
   d. petrous ridges.

4. The Lysholm method for imaging the skull base makes use of a _____ central ray angle.

   a. 37° caudad
   b. 35° caudad
   c. 37° cephalad
   d. 30° caudad

5. The OML forms a _____ angle to the film in the Waters method.

   a. 15°
   b. 10°
   c. 30°
   d. 37°

6. A PA projection with the head positioned MSP and the OML perpendicular to the film demonstrates the petrous ridges

   a. in the lower one-third of the orbits.
   b. below the orbits.
   c. filling the orbits.
   d. below the maxillary sinuses.

7. The paranasal sinuses are best imaged with the patient erect in order to demonstrate

   a. air-fluid levels.
   b. true size.
   c. septum disease.
   d. air pressure.

8. The sphenoidal sinuses are best seen when the patient is positioned for a _____ projection.

   a. AP
   b. SMV
   c. AP axial
   d. Townes

9. In an AP axial projection (Towne method), with the IOML perpendicular to the film, the central ray should be directed

   a. 30° caudad.
   b. 25° caudad.
   c. 37° caudad.
   d. 5° cephalad.

10. Rotate the head _____ for an oblique tangential projection of a zygomatic arch.

    a. 15° away from the affected side
    b. 45° toward the affected side
    c. 15° toward the affected side
    d. 45° away from the affected side

11. When the parietoorbital oblique position (Rhese method) is used properly, the optic foramen can be seen in the
    a. upper outer quadrant.
    b. lower one-third of the orbits.
    c. maxillary sinuses.
    d. lower outer quadrant.

12. The central ray is directed _____ in the Mayer method.
    a. 25° caudad
    b. 45° caudad
    c. 10° cephalad
    d. 30° caudad

13. The PA axial position (Haas method) is comparable to the
    a. Waters method.
    b. AP axial position.
    c. SMV position.
    d. Schuller method.

14. An anterior profile projection (Arcelin method) makes use of a _____ central ray angle.
    a. 10° caudad
    b. 10° cephalad
    c. 12° caudad
    d. 12° cephalad

15. For a lateral skull projection the head is adjusted so that the _____ is parallel to the film.
    a. coronal plane
    b. MML
    c. MSP
    d. IPL

16. A name given to the point where the nasal septum and the upper lip meet is the
    a. glabella.
    b. mentum.
    c. gonion.
    d. acanthion.

17. The position or projection that demonstrates *all* the sinuses on one film is the
    a. SMV.
    b. lateral.
    c. Waters.
    d. Caldwell.

18. The outer junction of the eyelids is called the
    a. inner canthus.
    b. EAM.
    c. outer canthus.
    d. TEA.

19. The central ray location for a lateral sella turcica is _____ to the EAM.

    a. ¾ in. anterior and inferior
    b. 2 in. superior
    c. 2 in. anterior and superior
    d. ¾ in. anterior and superior

20. The difference between the OML and the IOML is

    a. 12°.
    b. 10°.
    c. 7°.
    d. 8°.

21. A parietoorbital oblique projection of the optic foramen requires the MSP to be _____ to the film.

    a. 37°
    b. 53°
    c. 23°
    d. 15°

22. A smooth, slightly depressed area at a midpoint above the eyebrows is known as the

    a. glabella.
    b. gonion.
    c. inion.
    d. nasion.

23. There is a _____ difference between the IOML and the GML.

    a. 7°
    b. 8°
    c. 12°
    d. 15°

24. A lateral position of the skull, sinuses, and facial bones requires the _____ to be perpendicular to the film.

    a. EAM
    b. IPL
    c. MSP
    d. AML

25. Reid's baseline is a name given to the

    a. IPL.
    b. OML.
    c. IOML.
    d. MSP.

26. The Caldwell method (PA axial position) requires a central ray direction of _____ to the OML.

    a. 15° caudad
    b. 15° cephalad
    c. 10° caudad
    d. 23° cephalad

27. Place the _____ parallel to the film when positioning the patient for a SMV projection.

    a. MSP
    b. OML
    c. IOML
    d. IPL

28. A modified Waters method places the OML 55° to the film, demonstrating the

    a. mastoids.
    b. orbital floors.
    c. petrous ridges.
    d. cranium.

29. Nasal bones are typically imaged

    a. bilaterally.
    b. obliquely.
    c. in the SMV position.
    d. unilaterally.

30. When the TMJs are imaged using the lateral transfacial position (Albers-Schonberg method), direct the central ray

    a. 25° caudad.
    b. 37° caudad.
    c. 30° cephalad.
    d. 29° caudad.

Gastrointestinal Tract

ESOPHAGRAM (BARIUM SWALLOW)

- An exposure is usually taken while the patient is drinking barium contrast in order to ensure complete esophageal filling.

- The esophagus is well demonstrated between the vertebrae and the heart in the 35 to 40° RAO position.

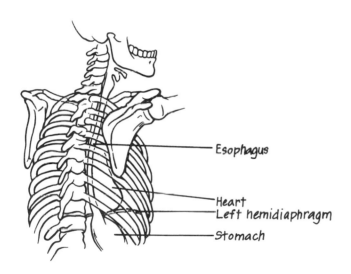

Esophagus

Heart
Left hemidiaphragm
Stomach

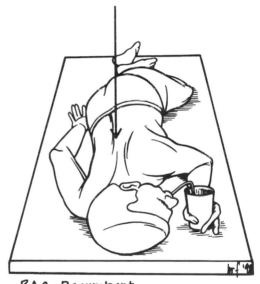

RAO - Recumbent

- A PA or AP projection (frontal image) demonstrates the esophagus superimposed over the T-spine.

- If the patient cannot lie semiprone in a RAO esophagus position, use an alternative LPO position.

UPPER GASTROINTESTINAL SERIES

- A PA projection of the stomach shows barium in the body and pylorus.

- An AP stomach image shows the concentration of barium in the fundus and duodenum.

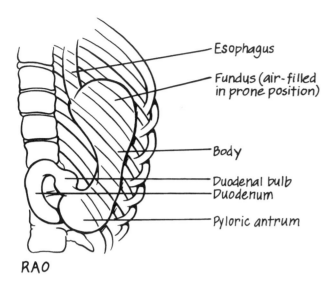

Esophagus

Fundus (air-filled in prone position)

Body

Duodenal bulb
Duodenum

Pyloric antrum

RAO

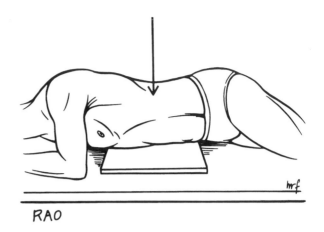

RAO

- A 40 to 70° RAO stomach projection best demonstrates the pyloric canal and the duodenal bulb.

- The central ray is directed toward L2 and is midway between the vertebral column and the left lateral abdominal border in an RAO stomach projection.

- If the patient cannot tolerate the semiprone position (RAO), use a 30 to 60° LPO position.

- A right lateral position demonstrates the anterior and posterior aspects of the stomach as well as the pyloric canal and duodenal bulb.

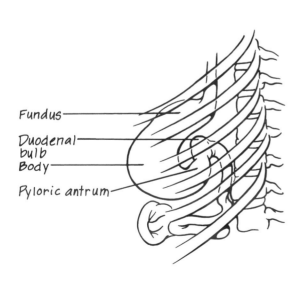

Fundus

Duodenal bulb
Body

Pyloric antrum

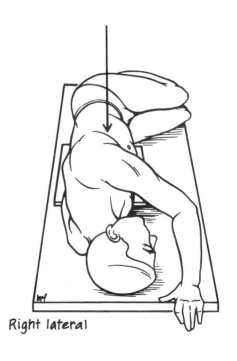

Right lateral

- An AP position with the table partially tilted (Trendelenburg position) and the head down may help to facilitate the demonstration of a hiatal hernia.

SMALL BOWEL SERIES

- Films are taken at timed intervals after barium is ingested, and fluoroscopy utilized when the barium reaches the terminal ileum (ileocecal valve).

- The preferred position for a small bowel examination is lying prone (PA) in order to naturally compress, spread, and separate the loops for improved viewing.

BARIUM ENEMA

- The 35 to 45° RAO position best shows the right colic (hepatic) flexure, cecum, the ascending colon, and sigmoid colon.

- A 35 to 45° LAO position demonstrates the splenic (left colic) flexure and the descending colon).

- A 35 to 45° LPO position demonstrates anatomy similar to that seen with a RAO position (hepatic flexure and the sigmoid colon).

- A 35 to 45° RPO position best demonstrates the splenic flexure (similarly to the LAO position).

- The central ray location for a left lateral rectum image is at the ASIS and midaxillary plane (MAL).

- An elongated view of the rectosigmoid region is achieved with the
  1. AP axial projection, 30 to 40° cephalad angle
  2. PA axial projection, 30 to 40° caudad angle
  3. 30 to 40° LPO projection, 30 to 40° cephalad angle.

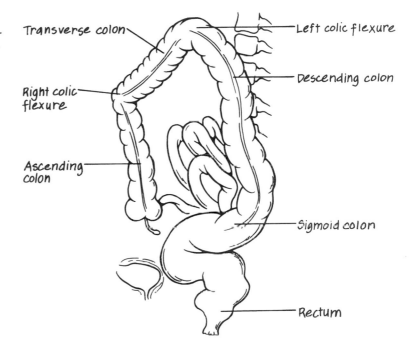

Transverse colon — Left colic flexure

Descending colon

Right colic flexure

Ascending colon

Sigmoid colon

Rectum

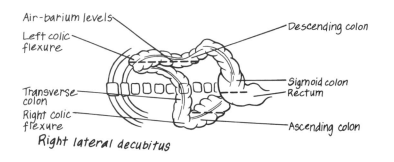

Air-barium levels
Left colic flexure
Descending colon
Transverse colon
Sigmoid colon
Rectum
Right colic flexure
Ascending colon

Right lateral decubitus

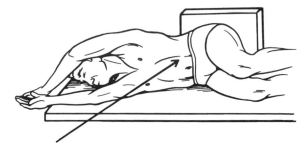

Right lateral decubitus position

- Decubitus positions are employed when the colon is examined using a double contrast (barium and air). The air rises and gravity pulls the barium downward for these images.

GALLBLADDER

- An oral cholecystogram (OCG) can be obtained in the radiology department to evaluate for gallstones.

- At least one image during an OCG examination should be taken with the patient upright or recumbent and using a horizontal central ray in order to better differentiate pathology.

- A 15 to 40° LAO film or an alternative 15 to 40° RPO film is taken with the central ray centered toward the midpoint of the right upper quadrant.

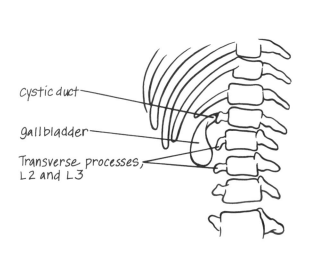

Cystic duct
gallbladder
Transverse processes, L2 and L3

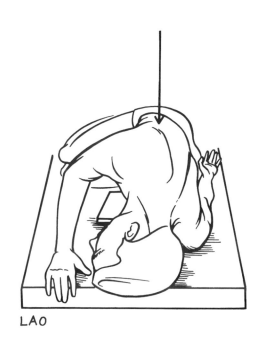

LAO

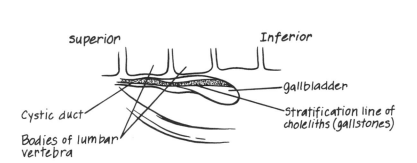

superior   Inferior

gallbladder

Cystic duct

Stratification line of choleliths (gallstones)

Bodies of lumbar vertebra

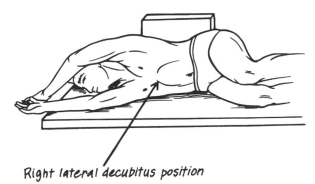

Right lateral decubitus position

- If a decubitus film is necessary, it must be a right lateral decubitus versus a left.

Chapter 8 Practice Questions

1. For demonstration of an open hepatic flexure during a BE examination this position is used.

   a. RPO
   b. RAO
   c. left lateral
   d. LAO

2. The Trendelenburg position is employed for an upper gastrointestinal series to help demonstrate

   a. the fundus.
   b. the greater curvature.
   c. motility.
   d. reflux and/or a hiatal hernia.

3. The esophagus is seen between the vertebrae and the heart in which position?

   a. AP
   b. PA
   c. 35 to 40° RAO
   d. 35 to 40° RPO

4. The central ray is directed at the _____ level for an RAO stomach image.

   a. L2
   b. L4
   c. T12
   d. T7

5. During an upper gastrointestinal series, visualization of an air-filled fundus and duodenum is accomplished with _____ position.

    a. an AP
    b. a RAO
    c. a PA
    d. a semiprone

6. Timed films of the small bowel are taken until barium reaches the

    a. duodenum.
    b. pylorus.
    c. ileocecal valve.
    d. cardiac valve.

7. The anterior and posterior aspects of the stomach are well visualized with the _____ position.

    a. left lateral
    b. RPO
    c. LPO
    d. right lateral

8. Natural compression and separation of the small bowel occur when the patient is in which position?

    a. supine
    b. prone
    c. upright
    d. decubitus

9. A _____ decubitus position may be necessary when the gallbladder is being imaged.

    a. ventral
    b. dorsal
    c. left lateral
    d. right lateral

10. Decubitus positions during a BE examination are used to evaluate

    a. barium uptake.
    b. single-contrast examinations.
    c. the intestinal lumen.
    d. gallstones.

11. An ideal barium swallow film demonstrates the esophagus

    a. filled with barium.
    b. in motion.
    c. over the spine.
    d. empty.

12. An alternative position for imaging an RAO esophagus is

    a. 60° LPO.
    b. 40° LPO.
    c. 60° RPO.
    d. AP.

13. An AP stomach image demonstrates the concentration of barium in the

    a. pylorus.
    b. body.
    c. fundus.
    d. esophagus.

14. The splenic flexure is seen free of overlap in the _____ position.

    a. 35 to 45° LAO
    b. 60° LAO
    c. 35 to 45° RAO
    d. 60° RAO

15. An OCG examination requires contrast to be administered

    a. intrathecally.
    b. intravenously.
    c. rectally.
    d. orally.

16. A right lateral decubitus BE film shows air "up" in the _____ colon.

    a. right flexure
    b. descending
    c. rectum
    d. ascending

17. The preferred oblique position for an OCG examination is

    a. 60° LAO.
    b. 60° RPO.
    c. 60° RAO.
    d. 30° LAO.

18. An RAO stomach position is recommended using _____ of obliquity.

    a. 30°
    b. 25°
    c. 60°
    d. 90°

19. The central ray location for a lateral rectum image is the

    a. IC and the MSP.
    b. IC and the MCP.
    c. ASIS and the MAL.
    d. ASIS and the MSP.

20. A PA axial projection of the rectosigmoid region employs a central ray direction of

    a. 30 to 40° caudad.
    b. 30 to 40° cephalad.
    c. 20° caudad.
    d. 60° cephalad.

Urinary System

- The **urinary system** consists of the kidneys, ureters, bladder, and urethra.

- **Intravenous urography (pyelography) (IVP)** is the study of the functions of the urinary system after the introduction of contrast.

- Ureteric compression can be used during IVP to help better demonstrate the renal collecting system and the proximal ureters.

- **Retrograde urography** is the nonfunctional study of the urinary system usually performed in the operating room under sterile conditions.

- **Retrograde cystography** is the nonfunctional study of only the urinary bladder.

- A **voiding cystourethrography (VCUG)** study is considered functional and is used to evaluate the patient's ability to urinate.

- An AP projection (scout or KUB) must include all of the urinary system with the symphysis pubis at the bottom of the collimated field.

- An AP nephrogram film is centered to include only the kidneys and a small portion of the proximal ureters.

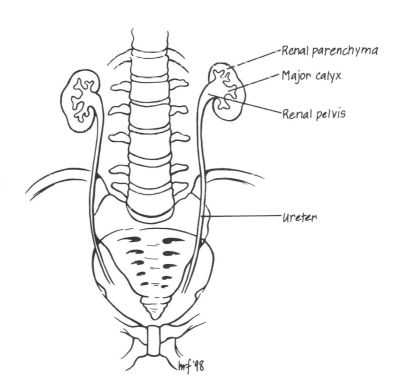

Renal parenchyma
Major calyx
Renal pelvis

Ureter

mf '98

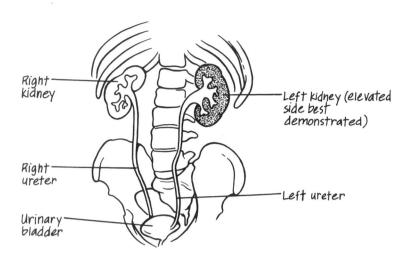

Right kidney

Left kidney (elevated side best demonstrated)

Right ureter

Left ureter

Urinary bladder

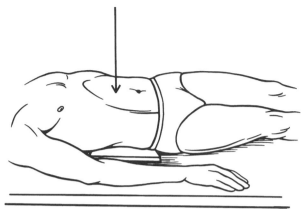

30° RPO (right AP oblique) position

- 30° posterior oblique (AP oblique) positions demonstrate the elevated side of the kidney in profile.

- An erect postvoid position helps to demonstrate nephroptosis and/or an enlarged prostate gland.

- An alternative position to the erect postvoid position is the prone (PA), if the patient's condition warrants.

- Posterior oblique positions of the bladder are recommended at a steepness of 45 to 60°.

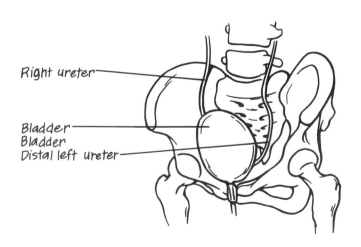

Right ureter

Bladder
Bladder
Distal left ureter

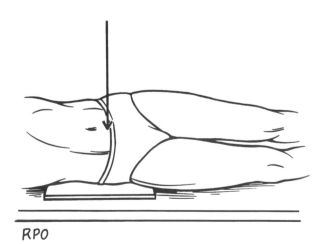

RPO

Chapter 9 Practice Questions

1. The urinary system consists of the

   1. kidneys.
   2. gallbladder.
   3. urethra.
   4. pancreas.

   a. 1 and 2
   b. 1, 2, and 3
   c. 1 and 3
   d. all of the above

2. An AP nephrogram film includes the

   a. bladder.
   b. kidneys.
   c. urethra.
   d. UV junction.

3. An RPO KUB projection demonstrates the _____ in profile.

   a. left IC
   b. right kidney
   c. left kidney
   d. left ureter

4. The degree of steepness recommended for an oblique bladder projection is

   a. 45 to 60°.
   b. 60 to 70°.
   c. 15 to 20°.
   d. 35 to 40°.

5. When better visualization or filling of the upper urinary system is desired, _____ can be used.

   a. relaxation
   b. VCUG
   c. a KUB
   d. compression

6. The structure that must be included for a complete KUB is the

   a. heart.
   b. hip joint.
   c. symphysis pubis.
   d. diaphragm.

7. The required degree of obliquity required for a nephrogram is

   a. 30°.
   b. 37°.
   c. 45°.
   d. 60°.

8. An erect postvoid position is ideal, however, if the patient is unable to stand, place him or her in the _____ position.

   a. supine
   b. prone
   c. 45° oblique
   d. 60° oblique

9. A VCUG study is considered to be
   a. functional.
   b. nonfunctional.
   c. useless.
   d. stressful.

10. A 30° LAO nephrogram demonstrates the _____ in profile.
    a. left ureter
    b. right kidney
    c. left kidney
    d. bladder

Special Examinations

- **Mammography** is the practice of imaging the breast tissue.

- An **operative cholangiogram** is an image taken in the surgical suite directly following a cholecystectomy.

- **T-tube cholangiography** involves imaging a special T-shaped catheter which is placed in a patient's common bile duct postoperatively.

- **Percutaneous transhepatic cholangiography (PTC)** involves imaging the biliary system after a needle puncture has been made through the liver and into the biliary ducts for the injection of contrast medium.

- An **endoscopic retrograde cholangiopancreatography (ERCP)** examination involves passing a scope through the mouth and stomach and into the duodenum for catheterization of the biliary system. Once this system is catheterized and contrast is successfully injected, images are taken of the biliary system.

- The study of the salivary glands using contrast medium is termed **sialography**.

- An **enteroclysis** procedure allows study of the small bowel following the injection of contrast medium through a nasogastric (NG) tube.

- **Metallic bead chain cystourethrography** is a method of investigating urinary stress incontinence problems in females.

- **Vesiculography, epididymography,** and **prostatography** are all examples of male reproductive system examinations.

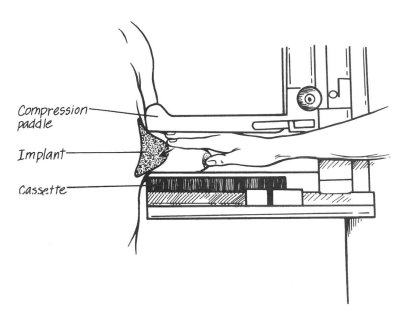

Compression paddle

Implant

Cassette

- **Hysterosalpingography** is the study of the female uterus and fallopian tubes.

- **Pelvimetry** and **cephalometry** are radiographic methods for measuring the pelvis and/or the head of the fetus in a pregnant patient using a special ruler (a Colcher-Sussman ruler).

- The **Sweet method** and the **Pfeiffer-Comberg method** make use of special apparatuses to localize intraorbital or intraocular foreign bodies.

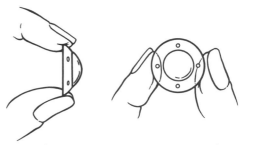

Pfeiffer-Comberg contact lens localization device

- Examination of the nasolacrimal ducts is accomplished using **dacryocystography**.

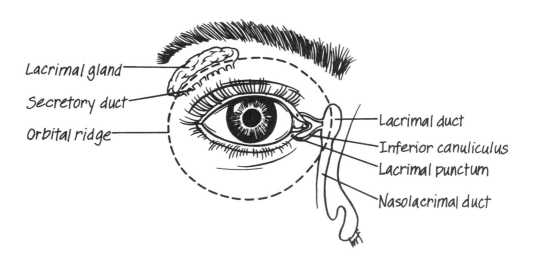

- **Orthoroentgenography** is a term used to describe a method of taking long bone measurements.

- A contrast media study of the synovial joints and related soft tissue is called **arthrography**.

- **Myelography** is an attempt to study the spinal cord and its nerve branches after introduction of intrathecal contrast medium.

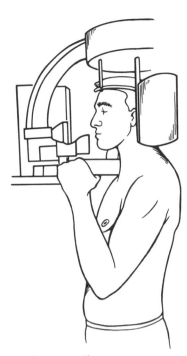

Panorex unit

- Conventional **tomography** is a means of obtaining body section images while blurring out structures above and below the objective tissue.

- **Computed tomography** (CT) differs from conventional tomography in that a computer processes, manipulates, and reconstructs the image.

- Radiographic examination of contrast-enhanced blood vessels is termed **angiography**.

- **Magnetic resonance imaging** (MRI) utilizes *no* x-rays. Rather it constructs images using magnetic fields and radio waves.

- An **ultrasound image** is formed by precise measurements of how sound waves react to the targeted tissues.

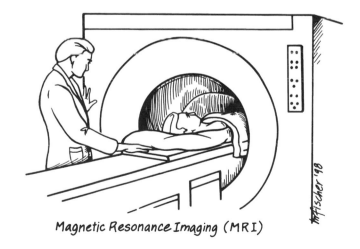

Magnetic Resonance Imaging (MRI)

Chapter 10 Practice Questions

1. A Colcher-Sussman ruler is used for examination of the
   a. ureters.
   b. spinal cord.
   c. tear ducts.
   d. fetus.

2. MRI equipment uses _____ energy to construct an image.
   a. x-ray
   b. sound
   c. light
   d. magnetic and radio wave

3. The study of breast tissue is accomplished by the use of
   a. dacryocystography.
   b. mammography.
   c. angiography.
   d. myelography.

4. Sialography is the radiographic study of the
   a. tear ducts.
   b. gallbladder.
   c. salivary glands.
   d. fallopian tubes.

5. The Sweet and Pfeiffer-Comberg methods help to localize foreign bodies in
   a. the eye.
   b. soft tissue.
   c. the trachea.
   d. the mouth.

6. Radiographic study of synovial joints is called
   a. sialography.
   b. myelography.
   c. arthrography.
   d. vesiculography.

7. A postoperative examination of the biliary system via a special catheter is called
   a. enteroclysis.
   b. PTC.
   c. myography.
   d. T-tube cholangiography.

8. **The small bowel can be studied after injection of contrast through a NG tube. This examination is called**

   a. hysterosalpingography.
   b. PTC.
   c. enteroclysis.
   d. sialography.

9. **Metallic bead chain cystourethrography is performed on a**

   a. male.
   b. female.
   c. fetus.
   d. breast.

10. **Myelography is the study of the _____ using contrast medium.**

   a. ventricles
   b. brain
   c. spinal cord
   d. heart

Appendices

Glossary

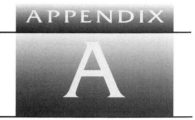

Abduction   Movement of a body part away from the midsagittal plane.

Acanthion   A radiographic landmark located at the junction of the nasal septum and upper lip.

Acute abdominal series (AAS)   A series of images (often called a three-way abdomen) consisting of a KUB (kidneys, ureters, bladder) image, an erect abdomen film, and a postero-anterior chest x-ray.

Adduction   Movement of a body part toward the midsagittal plane.

Albers-Schonberg method   A lateral transfacial projection used to demonstrate the temporomandibular joints.

Anatomical position   An erect body position with palms forward, feet together, and arms at the sides. Radiographs are typically displayed (viewed) in the anatomical position.

Anterior   Referring to the front or forward part of the body.

Anteroposterior (AP) projection   A projection in which the x-ray beam travels from the front to the back of the patient's body.

Arcelin method   An anterior projection that produces a profile of the petrous bone (reverse of the Stenvers method).

Axial plane   A horizontal plane dividing the body into superior and inferior portions.

Axial projection   An angled central ray directed through the long axis of the patient's body.

Ball catcher position   A bilateral anteroposterior oblique position of the hands used for demonstrating rheumatoid arthritis.

Beclere method   An anteroposterior axial projection of the intercondylar fossa with 30 to 40° knee flexion.

Body habitus   A term used to describe various body sizes and shapes.

Caldwell method   A posteroanterior axial projection for head work requiring a 15° caudad angle.

Camp Coventry method   A postero-anterior 40 to 50° axial projection of the intercondylar fossa with the knee flexed and the patient lying prone.

Carpal bridge projection   A tangential position of the wrist in extreme palmar flexion demonstrating the dorsal aspect of the carpal bones.

Carpal canal (tunnel) position   A tangential position of the hyperextended wrist allowing for the evaluation of carpal tunnel syndrome.

Caudad (caudal)   Describing a central ray direction toward the feet.

Cephalad (cephalic)   Describing a central ray direction toward the head.

Chassard-Lapine method   An axial pelvis position demonstrating the acetabulum and pelvimetry dimensions.

Clements-Nakayama method   A modified axiolateral projection of a traumatized hip.

Coronal plane   A vertical plane dividing the body into anterior and posterior portions.

Coyle method   An axiolateral projection of the elbow demonstrating the radial head and/or the coronoid process.

Danelius-Miller method   An axiolateral projection of a traumatized hip.

Decubitus position   A recumbent body position (lateral, ventral, or dorsal) requiring the use of a horizontal central ray.

Dorsal   Referring to the back portion of the body.

Dorsal decubitus position   A supine patient position requiring a horizontal central ray.

Dorsiflexion   The act of flexing the top of the foot upward.

Erect position   A standing or seated upright body position.

Eversion   Application of an outward movement or stress to a body part.

Extension   The act of straightening or increasing the angle of a joint or the spine.

Fan lateral position   A true lateral position of the hand with the digits slightly flexed and separated. This position provides optimal demonstration of the entire hand with minimal digit superimposition.

Flexion   The act of bending or decreasing the angle of a joint or the spine.

Fowler's position   A recumbent body position in which the head is higher than the feet.

Frog-leg hip position   A lateral position of the hip with the knee flexed and the thigh abducted 40 to 45° from the vertical (modified Cleaves method).

Frontal plane   A vertical plane dividing the body into anterior and posterior portions.

Fuchs method   An anteroposterior projection with the chin extended used in demonstrating the dens within the foramen magnum.

Glabella   A radiographic landmark located between the eyebrows.

Gonion   The angle of the mandible.

Grashey method   An anteroposterior oblique position of the shoulder used in demonstrating the glenohumeral joint.

Haas method   A posteroanterior axial projection yielding information similar to that obtained from the Towne method. The central ray is directed 25° cephalad.

Henschen method   An axiolateral head work projection utilizing a 15° caudad central ray angle.

Holmblad method   A posteroanterior axial projection of the intercondylar fossa with the knee flexed approximately 70°.

Hughston method   A tangential projection of the patella while the patient is prone.

Hypersthenic   A massive-build body habitus with high, transverse organ placement.

Hyposthenic (asthenic)   A small, thin body type typically with long, narrow organs placed relatively low in the body cavities.

Inferosuperior axial position (Lawrence method)   A supine position with the affected arm abducted 90° and the central ray directed through the axilla used in demonstrating the glenohumeral joint.

Intercondylar fossa   The space between the condyles of the femur.

Inversion   Application of an inward movement or stress to a specific body part.

Judd method   A posteroanterior projection of the dens with the chin extended to place the orbitomeatal line 37° to the film plane.

Kite method   A technique of imaging the foot in its natural position for the evaluation of congenital clubfoot (talipes equinovarus).

Lateral   A body position that produces a side view of a specific body part.

Law method   An axiolateral oblique projection of the head used to demonstrate various structures.

Lawrence method   A transthoracic position used to demonstrate the proximal third of the lateral humerus. (See also inferosuperior axial position.)

Leonard-George method   An axiolateral projection of a traumatized hip.

Lithotomy position   A supine body position with the knees flexed, thighs abducted, and legs placed on supports.

Lordotic chest projection   An anteroposterior projection of the chest either while the patient leans back or with a cephalic central ray angle in order to demonstrate the apical chest region.

Lysholm method   A true lateral position of the skull utilizing a 35° caudad central ray angle.

Mayer method   An axioposterior oblique position with the head rotated 45° utilizing a 45° caudad central ray angle.

Merchant method   A method of imaging bilateral patellas using a preset leg angling device.

Method   A radiographic position or projection named after the person who developed it.

Midcoronal plane   A vertical plane dividing the body into equal front and back portions.

Midsagittal plane   A vertical midline plane dividing the body into equal right and left halves.

Mortise view   A 15 to 20° internal oblique position of the ankle best demonstrating the mortise joint.

Nasion   A radiographic landmark at the junction of the nasal and frontal bones.

Oblique   A rotated body position in which neither a frontal or lateral image is produced.

Open mouth odontoid   A method of imaging the odontoid process (dens) through a patient's open mouth.

Ottonello method   An anteroposterior or entire C-spine projection during intentional jaw movement (wagging jaw method).

Owen method   A modified Mayer method requiring a 30 to 40° head rotation and a 30 to 40° caudad central ray angle.

Panorex (orthopantomogram)   A panoramic view (radiograph) of the entire mandible.

Pawlow method   A recumbent swimmer's lateral position.

Pirie method   An axial transoral position for demonstrating the sphenoid sinuses.

Plantar flexion   The act of extending the foot downward.

Position   The body placement of a patient relative to the film or surrounding space.

Posterior   Referring to the back portion of the body.

Posteroanterior (PA) projection   A projection in which the x-ray beam travels from the back to the front of the patient's body.

Projection   The direction or path of the x-ray beam as it passes through the patient.

Prone   A position in which the patient is lying face down; the opposite of supine.

Radiograph An x-ray film with a manifest anatomical image.

Recumbent Any body position in which the patient is lying down.

Reid's baseline A formal name given to the infraorbitomeatal line.

Rhese method A parietoorbital projection (posteroanterior) demonstrating the downside (dependent) orbit when the patient's chin, cheek, and nose are resting on the image receptor.

Sagittal plane A vertical plane dividing the body into right and left portions.

Schuller method An axiolateral (transcranial) projection used for head work.

Settegast (sunrise) A tangential projection of the patella while the patient is supine with the knee flexed.

Stecher method A wrist position in which an angled part or central ray allows for improved visualization of the carpal navicular (scaphoid).

Stenvers method An axiolateral oblique (posterior profile) with the head resting on the forehead, cheek, and nose.

Sthenic Referring to an average-build body habitus.

Supine A position in which the patient is lying on the back.

Swimmer's position A positioning method in which the patient is in the lateral position with one arm raised and one arm lowered used in demonstrating the cervicothoracic junction.

Tangential projection A central ray projection that "skims" the body part of interest.

Towne method An anteroposterior 30° angle projection utilized for head work.

Transverse plane A horizontal plane dividing the body into superior and inferior portions.

Trendelenburg position A recumbent body position with the table angled to place the feet higher than the head.

Twining method An upright swimmer's lateral method used in demonstrating the cervicothoracic region.

Ventral Referring to the front or forward part of the body.

Ventral decubitus position A prone patient position requiring a horizontal central ray.

Waters method A parietoacanthial projection with the orbitomeatal line 37° to the film.

Y position An oblique (usually 60°) position of the shoulder which is useful in the evaluation of suspected shoulder dislocations.

Bibliography

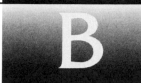

Ballinger PW. *Merrill's Atlas of Radiographic Positions and Radiologic Procedures.* Mosby, St. Louis, 1991, vol. 1, pp. 36–455; vol. 2, pp. 15–447; vol. 3, pp. 24–357.

Ballinger PW. *Pocket Guide to Radiography.* Mosby, St. Louis, 1995.

Bontrager KL. *Pocket Handbook of Radiographic Positioning and Techniques.* Bontrager, Ariz., 1995.

Bontrager KL. *Textbook of Radiographic Positioning and Related Anatomy.* Mosby, St. Louis, 1997.

Cornuelle AG, Gronefeld DH. *Radiographic Anatomy and Positioning: An Integrated Approach.* Appleton & Lange, Norwalk, Conn., 1998, pp. 46–547.

Cullinan, AM. *Optimizing Radiographic Positioning.* JB Lippincott, Philadelphia, 1992, pp. 24–223.

Dowd SB, Wilson BG. *Encyclopedia of Radiographic Positioning.* WB Saunders, Philadelphia, 1995, vol. 1, pp. 109–521; vol. 2, pp. 525–1151.

Eisenberg RL, Dennis CA, May CR. *Radiographic Positioning.* Little, Brown, Boston, 1995, pp. 11–385.

Hagler, MJ. *The Pocket Rad Tech.* WB Saunders, Philadelphia, 1993.

Answers
to Practice Questions

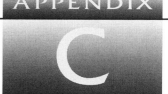

Chapter 1
1. c
2. d
3. b
4. d
5. b
6. b
7. d
8. a
9. a
10. d
11. b
12. c
13. c
14. d
15. c
16. b
17. b
18. c
19. a
20. b
21. b
22. d
23. c
24. b
25. b
26. d
27. b
28. d
29. a
30. b

Chapter 2
1. a
2. b
3. c
4. d
5. d
6. b
7. c
8. b
9. c

10. a
11. c
12. c
13. d
14. b
15. a
16. c
17. b
18. b
19. a
20. c
21. d
22. a
23. b
24. d
25. b
26. c
27. a
28. c
29. c
30. a

Chapter 3
1. a
2. d
3. b
4. b
5. c
6. c
7. a
8. d
9. a
10. c
11. b
12. a
13. b
14. a
15. c
16. b
17. a
18. c
19. d

20. b
21. c
22. d
23. a
24. d
25. c
26. b
27. b
28. c
29. b
30. c

Chapter 4
1. c
2. b
3. b
4. b
5. a
6. d
7. a
8. c
9. c
10. b
11. a
12. d
13. b
14. d
15. c
16. b
17. c
18. a
19. a
20. b

Chapter 5
1. b
2. c
3. d
4. c
5. a
6. b
7. b

8. c
9. a
10. b

Chapter 6
1. b
2. c
3. d
4. c
5. c
6. a
7. b
8. d
9. d
10. a
11. c
12. c
13. d
14. b
15. c
16. a
17. a
18. d
19. b
20. c
21. b
22. c
23. b
24. a
25. d
26. b
27. c
28. a
29. c
30. a

Chapter 7
1. c
2. b

3. a
4. b
5. d
6. c
7. a
8. b
9. c
10. c
11. d
12. b
13. b
14. a
15. c
16. d
17. b
18. c
19. d
20. c
21. b
22. a
23. d
24. b
25. c
26. a
27. c
28. b
29. a
30. d

Chapter 8
1. b
2. d
3. c
4. a
5. c
6. c
7. d
8. b
9. d

10. c
11. a
12. b
13. c
14. a
15. d
16. b
17. d
18. c
19. c
20. a

Chapter 9
1. c
2. b
3. c
4. a
5. d
6. c
7. a
8. b
9. a
10. c

Chapter 10
1. d
2. d
3. b
4. c
5. a
6. c
7. d
8. c
9. b
10. c

ISBN 0-07-058067-7

90000

9 780070 580671

SCHUBERT: PATIENT
POSITIONING